The Parenting Journey:
Raising Deaf and Hard of Hearing Children

by Karen Putz

Copyright © 2012 by Karen Putz

Barefoot Publications

www.karenputz.com

For David, Lauren and Steven,
you light up my world.

To everyone who has crossed my path,
thank you. You enriched the journey.

Welcome to the Journey

Let your mind start a journey through a strange new world. Leave all thoughts of the world you knew before. Let your soul take you where you long to be... Close your eyes let your spirit start to soar, and you'll live as you've never lived before.

~Erich Fromm

Welcome to the journey of life with deaf and hard of hearing kids.

This book chronicles my own journey. I have three kids, a hubby, and a cute West Highland White Terrier. I once tried to claim them all on a tax form but apparently the government has a definition of a "dependent" that is a bit different from mine.

I'm deaf, I'm a mom of three deaf and hard of hearing kids, and I also work as a Deaf Mentor in early intervention. I work with families from birth to age three, answering questions and providing information and resources. I've been on the other end of the service spectrum as well. Steven, my youngest kiddo, received early intervention services when he was a toddler.

David is my oldest and he is now a young adult. Every time I try to call him-- *David, Daaavid, DAVID!* --he doesn't always respond. I don't know if it is because he has his eyes glued to the computer or if it is because he has a very low line on his audiogram. From the time he was little, he was the original Energizer Bunny. Long after I flung myself on the couch in defeat, he would keep going, going, going. And going.

Lauren is my middle child and she's the little girl I always dreamed of having. Unfortunately, when she was about three, she decided I could no longer dress her in pink bows and frilly dresses. She hated her pink room and demanded that I paint over it in blue and green. She wanted to be like her brothers and she frequently borrowed David's clothes. I was devastated. I waited all my life for a little girl and she was boycotting the girly image. I shouldn't have worried, because she now calls the mall her second home and owns 20 different colors of nail polish. We constantly fight about the dresses she wants to wear; I want them below her knees and she wants them above. And she has a pink room again. This time, she's covered the walls with inspirational quotes.

Steven is my youngest kiddo, the one who goes with the flow and never raises an argument. He's quick to lend a helping hand around the house and sometimes he surprises me by emptying the dishwasher without being told. He is happiest when he's glued to the computer, just like his brother. He always asks questions which make me think. He loves water sports and track. This kid was born at home, all nine-pounds of him.

My husband is also deaf. He is part of the Rubella generation of late 50's - early 60's, when a large number of children were born deaf or hard of hearing due to maternal Rubella. Joe was diagnosed at the age of three. He grew up in a neighborhood with several other deaf and hard of hearing kids, many who are his friends today.

I was born with normal hearing, diagnosed as hard of hearing when I was seven shortly after an illness with high fever. I became profoundly deaf at the age of nineteen from a fall while waterskiing on my bare feet. I'm from a family with five generations of hearing loss; all of us were born with normal hearing and became deaf or hard of hearing as a result of a rare genetic mutation that is passed on via the females in our family. To date, there are only two other families in the world who have been identified with the same gene. You can read more about my genetic story at my blog: www.karenputz.com.

I am a board member of Hands & Voices (www.handsandvoices.org), a parent-driven organization dedicated to providing support and information to families with deaf and hard of hearing children. I started the Illinois chapter and I serve on the board. I'm also the Coordinator of Deaf and Hard of Hearing Infusion. Today, Hands & Voices serves families worldwide.

Have I figured this parenting gig out? Heck no. But after packing a couple of parenting years under my belt, perhaps sharing what I've learned along the way might help you on your own journey. Maybe with some wise words of advice and a few chuckles, you might find that a few of your own parenting paths may smooth out as a result.

Some days are more challenging than others, but every step of the journey has been a lesson in learning. I have a lot more steps ahead of me to experience, but I've learned if you have others along in the journey, the path is so much richer as a result.

Enjoy the journey!

Chapter 1
How My Own Parenting Journey Began

Beginnings are usually scary and endings are usually sad, but it's the middle that counts. You have to remember this when you find yourself at the beginning.

~ Sandra Bullock

Back when David was two-years-old, I was involved in a parent group which provided support to parents with deaf and hard of hearing kids in the Chicago area. I volunteered my time with this group on a monthly basis. My background is in counseling, with my Masters degree in Rehabilitation Counseling so I always loved helping others.

One night, I was asked to lead the group and the parents began to talk about their feelings. There was a lot of sharing going on, a few tears, questions about communication modes, questions about cochlear implants and hearing aids. I did my best to try and connect with the parents and empathize with them, but I had no personal experience to drawn on as a parent.

Little did I know, a few short weeks later, my own parenting journey down the same road was about to begin. David was exhibiting signs (no pun intended, of course) his sense of hearing wasn't what it used to be. I began to suspect he lost some of his hearing. It took several weeks of arguing with the HMO pediatrician to convince the doctor of the need for a hearing test. He tried to reassure me by testing with a tuning fork and calling David's name. Of course, the kid turned to look at him and the doctor berated me for being an over-concerned mom. I left the office in tears, but I persisted in calling his office and asking for a referral to the local hospital. After I finally wrestled the referral from the reluctant physician, it took another several weeks to get an appointment at the hospital to schedule an ABR (Auditory Brainstem Response) hearing test.

David wasn't an easy kid to sedate. He was my "Energizer Bunny" child, and true to form, he fought off sleep. It took a Herculean effort to keep him from climbing out of the bed while we waited for the sedatives to kick in. Once he finally conked out, the audiologist hooked up the machine and we sat and watched. She began to record responses on the computer.

I saw a few 70s pop up. A few 90s.

I knew.

I looked over at my husband and signed, "He's deaf." Of course, the hubby didn't trust my brilliant audiological skills which were honed by a mere semester of audiology in college.

"Let's wait for the results," he said. He looked away.

I began to pester the audiologist for answers the moment she got up from the chair after she finished the test. "It looks like a severe-to-profound loss. He's deaf, isn't he?"

Her eyes did not meet mine. "Let me just wrap up here and meet you in my office," she said.

I knew.

I don't remember much after that. I do remember the audiologist going over the audiogram results, explaining that yes, indeed, David had a severe-to-profound hearing loss. David sat in my lap, restless. He tugged at my shirt and tried to get down on the floor. He was ready to go home.
I tried to focus on the audiologist's words. The rest of what she said became a blur. Something about hearing aids, speech therapy, and follow up.

"Do you have any questions?"

We didn't. Yet, we did.

We were still absorbing this sudden change in our parenting path but we didn't know what to do next or what questions to ask. We made the appointment to come back and get fitted for hearing aids. Later, in the car, mulling over every aspect of the day, I realized how little support we received after the diagnosis. We were sent home with a folder containing information about hearing loss. There was no information on how to connect with other families. No binder of resources. No seasoned parent with words of wisdom to provide some guidance.

It was quiet between the two of us on the ride home. We tried to dissect the diagnosis of profound hearing loss and what it meant. David fell asleep in the car seat, exhausted from the whole experience. I know I shed some tears as Joe and I talked. I remember reflecting back on my own childhood and my husband was doing the same. On one hand, we knew our kid was going to be just fine. After all, the hubby and I had created a nice life together. We had a circle of friends who were deaf, hard of hearing and hearing. Life was full.

On the other hand, we knew the challenges ahead. We knew what it was like on a daily basis to navigate life minus the full sense of hearing--and we wondered and worried-- would our kid go through the same things?

Today is my second child's birthday. Choosing to have another child after Jordan was born profoundly deaf was an act of love. Time and again throughout our journey our love, patience and strength have been tested. Love, patience and strength have always persevered. We share our mishaps, bruises and painful cuts with an international community of families who navigate our same path, and we overcome those challenging moments together. The other day Jordan and Sofia were playing Dance Party 3 together, and I sat watching and laughing with them. My son won, and my daughter was so happy he had played with her. Deafness is only one aspect of our lives; it does not define us, but how we have chosen to live it, has enriched us.

~ Jodi Cutler, Italy

Chapter 2
Finding Support

**When you have come to the edge
of all the light you have
And step into the darkness of the unknown
Believe that one of the two will happen to you
Either you'll find something solid to stand on
Or you'll be taught how to fly!**

~ Richard Bach

Despite my many years of working with families with deaf and hard of hearing kids, I soon discovered it was a whole other ballgame to navigate life as a parent of a deaf child. I was fortunate I had a network of parents to connect with thanks to my previous work with the support group. Our days were filled with trips to the audiologist and the local center for speech therapy. The school district arranged for preschool with other deaf and hard of hearing kids. I visited the school with David and did my best to explain he would now be going there every day. There would be no more "all day" sessions hanging out with mom at home. I was grieving more about this than anything else. The school was located several towns away and would require a 45-minute drive.

I did not want to put my kid on a bus.

I shared my concerns with my mother-in-law and she tried to

put my apprehension to rest. "I put Joe on the bus when he was three," she said. "And he had a long ride—over an hour each way. I cried a lot in the beginning, but I felt it was the best thing for him. This is something you're just going to have to do for David."

So the first day I put David on the bus, I was a nervous wreck. How do you get a three-year-old to comprehend that he was about to embark on a long bus ride to hang with people he met once? I plastered a smile on my face as I watched the bus pull away. Then I sat on the couch and cried. And cried.

Some days were easier than others. Then we had a new bus driver who made me uneasy. I couldn't put my finger on it, but I just didn't trust the guy. That afternoon, he pulled up to the house and I spied a cigarette butt on the floor of the bus. The Mama Tiger in me came out. One call to the bus company and he was no longer bussing my kid; and we soon had an aide riding on the bus as well.

That first year of preschool was an unsettling one. I did not like the teacher at all—she was near retirement and she seemed stuck in the old ways of teaching and disciplining a child. Her vibe was not a positive one. The co-teacher was a much more comfortable fit in the classroom. But all of this was still so new to me and I wasn't at a point where I was confident enough to exercise my own choices. At the time, I felt like I was roped into just one option to be able to get services with other deaf and hard of hearing kids.

Life had settled into a routine when Lauren and Steven both became sick with a high fever. The illness lasted for about a week.   When Lauren returned home from preschool, she said, "Mom, I can't hear."

My heart stopped. This was the kid who spoke in complete sentences at 14-months of age. This was the kid who loved to talk on the phone with her grandma and her friends. Oh yeah, this was the kid who loved music.

A visit to the audiologist showed she had a moderate-to-severe loss. Somehow it was much harder to deal with the news than with David. Perhaps it was because she was older and she knew what she was missing out on. In any case, it was a loss for all of us. The Lauren we knew for the last four years had changed overnight and now we were on a new road together.

At the time, we qualified for a state program that covered hearing aids, but they would only cover analog hearing aids per the school audiologist's recommendation. I wanted to purchase the digital hearing aids from the private audiologist who was also enrolled in the state program. The state program refused to pay for the digital hearing aids, saying that if the school audiologist recommended the analog hearing aids, they would go with her opinion. I was furious. I called the director of the state program, but they wouldn't budge. We ended up paying for every penny of the digital hearing aids out of our pocket. Fortunately for us, the audiologist accepted a payment plan.

Lauren grieved, and she grieved hard. She cried openly for several days and I had to bite my tongue to keep from crying along with her. She hated the hearing aids and wanted nothing to do with them.

"I don't want to wear them!" She stomped her feet. She pulled the hearing aids out and threw them on the kitchen floor. "I want my hearing back!"

I didn't make an issue out of the hearing aids because everything was too fresh, too raw. There would be time for that challenge later.

It was especially heartbreaking when her best friend called her on the phone and she couldn't understand half of what was said. She threw the phone on the floor. Tears streamed down her face. "I can't hear her!" she wailed. I gave her a hug, fighting back my own tears. As she trotted off to the living room, I went into the bathroom, sat on the toilet... and cried.

I was so entrenched in helping Lauren to adjust to this new reality and I was deep into dealing with school issues for David--I forgot about my youngest kid. We took a trip to the pediatrician because we were concerned about his strange gait. One leg was shorter than the other, but the doctor reassured us that it would not be noticeable as he grew. A few months later, I realized Steven wasn't talking. Steven didn't pick up signing and he wanted nothing to do with any of the language activities that my older two enjoyed at his age. It was hard to get his attention. He had trouble looking at strangers and his interaction was limited, even with family members. At two and half, he had behaviors that were very different from my other two kids. I could not get him to sit still and read a book with me. He insisted on mac and cheese for lunch every day and refused to try any new foods.

The kid's speech and language skills were definitely delayed. You would think that the obvious thing to do would be to test his hearing, right?

Well, Denial isn't just a winding river in Egypt. It's a coping mechanism that is neatly packaged for parents who aren't ready to deal with *The Real World*. So what did I do? I ignored the problems a little longer. Then friends began to take notice and make comments. I finally called up my local early intervention office and rustled up some speech therapy services. Surely a little early intervention would take care of "the problem" and get him talking.

I was in the living room on the floor playing with Steven, when the speech therapist knocked on the door. Steven didn't look up. She looked at me and the first words out of her mouth were, "He's deaf! Have you had his hearing tested?"

So, off we trotted to the audiologist's office and came out with a fresh audiogram to add to the growing pile of paperwork that my kids were collecting. Steven had nearly the same numbers on the audiogram as Lauren.

Well, there went my "Mother of the Year" award. Despite five generations of deaf and hard of hearing folks in my family, I didn't recognize my son as one until someone else figured it out.

By this time, I was pretty overwhelmed. Never mind the fact that having three kids two years apart is pretty overwhelming—we now had regular visits with the Ear, Nose and Throat doctor, the audiologists, speech therapists and the IEP teams at different schools. Everyone had an opinion to add to the mix, and sometimes one piece of advice contradicted the other. In the midst of it all, my 14-year-old niece came to live with us and she started high school. She was carrying a lot of emotional baggage being a teen and I wasn't equipped to mother her in the way she needed to be mothered. I dropped a lot of balls at that time.

Speaking of balls, the jumble of feelings inside of me was like a bouncing rubber ball. The ball was filled with those words we're oh-so-familiar with: grief, denial, depression, anger. Other days, it would be acceptance, accomplishment and celebration. Sometimes the ball was bouncing off the walls at speeds faster than the eye. And sometimes the ball would settle down long enough so I could focus on other things. And then it would start bouncing again, sometimes wildly, sometimes rhythmically. And sometimes the ball would bounce for such a long time it was totally interfering with daily life.

I found myself struggling with the medical point of view which seemed so cut-and-dry compared to everything I had experienced since becoming deaf. I was finally in a place where I was comfortable with being deaf and now I was raising deaf and hard of hearing kids. You'd think I would know what to do, right? Every visit to the audiologist focused on the numbers on the audiogram, but I was longing for support and guidance.

A few years later, my experience with the medical system was the catalyst for me to explore the options that were out there for parents. I decided to develop a website for Illinois and put together all of the resources in one place. In the process of creating the website, I stumbled on Hands & Voices. My heart skipped a beat when I read the mission and vision:

Hands & Voices is dedicated to supporting families with children who are Deaf or Hard of Hearing without a bias around communication modes or methodology. We're a parent-driven, non-profit organization providing families with the resources, networks, and information they need to improve communication access and educational outcomes for their children. Our outreach activities, parent/professional collaboration, and advocacy efforts are focused on enabling Deaf and Hard-of-Hearing children to reach their highest potential.

This was me! This was exactly how I felt about deaf and hard of hearing children--that there was no one "right" way. I loved being able to speak and I loved to sign and there were times I used each exclusively and even times I mashed them together. I just wanted to be me and I needed a safe place to explore this new path. It's one thing to work as a professional in the field. It's another thing to be a deaf/hard of hearing person. And it was a whole other ballgame to step into the parenting journey as a mom of a deaf kid--times three.

"We all take different paths in life, but no matter where we go, we take a little of each other everywhere."

~ Tim McGraw

Raising Olivia

~ Jeanne Carlisle

Olivia was born at 34 weeks by an emergency C-section. She had to be delivered because I could not feel her moving around in my belly. The doctor had me go to the hospital and they confirmed something was wrong. Olivia was born with a red blood cell count of four instead of 15-20 like other babies. She needed a blood transfusion right away. We got to see her briefly and then she was taken off to the NICU.

Those first few days in the hospital we were bombarded with lots of different medical issues Olivia was experiencing. It took a few days before she was able to eat without a feeding tube, and keep food in. It was another day before they took off the oxygen tube.

Shortly after she was born they told us they expected Olivia to have to stay in the NICU until at least the day she was due to be delivered, five weeks away. However, Olivia kept improving faster than they expected. She was released from the hospital six days after she was born. (That should have been our first sign of how strong she was, and what a great fighter she would be.)

While we were in the NICU going over all the instructions for discharge, and all the test results they told us Olivia did not pass the Newborn Hearing test. They had performed it two different times, and she failed both times. We were told not to worry too much about it. That it happened many times to babies born like Olivia, and that it was usually due to fluid in the ears that would clear up in a few days. We knew about the kidney and liver damage from the blood loss, but until we were about to walk out of the hospital with our baby, no one told us she had failed the hearing tests.

We repeated the testing as instructed and Olivia still did not pass, so we went for an ABR when she was 6 weeks old. It was at that time that we found out Olivia was profoundly deaf in her left ear, there was no brain stem response to any sounds at any frequency, but she had "perfect hearing" in her right ear. The Audiologist told us with one good ear we really did not have to do anything special for Olivia.

No, she didn't need hearing aids. She would have problems with being able to detect where sounds came from, and that when she was school age she might need preferential seating near the teacher and maybe a microphone system from the teacher to a speaker on her desk as well, but otherwise that was it. She did tell us to follow up with an ENT she recommended. We saw him about two weeks later and he confirmed what the audiologist said. The only thing extra he added was have the test repeated when she was three months old.

This advice never sat well with me. It seemed we should be doing more for Olivia. But they were the experts right? We followed up and took Olivia in when she was three months old. We were very anxious that the tests would show something different. However, the equipment was not working.

The audiologist tried a few times to get it to work. She turned it on and off. She even tried changing her equipment with another set up from another audiologist, but she could not get it to work. She apologized a number of times, but we had to leave without the tests being done. The next available appointment was 5 weeks later. So we waited. It had to be in a different location, and I don't think the audiologist was as comfortable at the different location, but they only ran the test on her good right ear.

The audiologist told us there was no point in retesting the other ear since she was deaf in that ear. She did tell us we would hear from the ENT again after he reviewed the tests from that day.

After two and a half weeks of not hearing from the ENT, I picked up the phone and called his office. It took about two weeks more before the ENT and I got to talk over the phone, but this time I expressed my concern with only testing one ear, and with not doing anything for Olivia's bad ear. He explained a lot of different things, and when he used words I didn't understand I made him go back and explain it in a way I would understand. This was the first time I really felt like I was not going to just listen to them, to take notes and sit silently by as they told me what to do for my child. He did tell me he would recommend that we brought her in for a surgical ABR. That instead of just having her sleep through the test like before, they would be able to get better results running it this way.

When I called the Audiologist to schedule the test, she did not agree. She did not feel we needed to put a baby that young through the anesthesia. She told me we could do whatever we wanted, but she did not think it was necessary. *Great*. We were relying on these two people, as experts, to tell us what to do, and they did not agree on what that was.

My husband and I had to think about it long and hard. We talked about newborns who go in for open heart surgery one or two days after being born, and how often that happens. We knew that they weren't going to be operating on Olivia, and that no one was going to cut her open. She just had to receive the anesthesia so they could monitor her brain stem activity during the test. We decided it was better to go ahead with the test and get the info instead of wondering if things were the same or worse. The test was done within 20 minutes and Olivia did fine. It confirmed the loss in her left ear, but it showed a very slight change in the right ear. It had dropped a little, but was still in the normal hearing range. We were told to bring Olivia back when she turned one so they could check on her hearing. That was it. There was nothing else that they were going to do, and no one offered us any kind of help or support with Olivia. We were sent home to raise her.

When Olivia turned one two things happened. I took her in to her pediatrician for her one year check up, and I took her in for the follow up check on her hearing. The pediatrician checked her out and said she was good. He also let me know he had something for me that might help with Olivia. It was a flyer, and that I should make sure I got it before I left. I had to ask the nurse for it, since it was not given to us. She had to go track down the doctor to find out what he was talking about, but eventually they found the flyer for Early Intervention (EI) and I was on my way home. Within days Olivia had her hearing retested by the audiologist, and this time the tests showed a loss in her good ear. It was enough that they wanted to run the tests again on another day to make sure they were correct, and not just a one year old getting too tired to cooperate.

Before we could run the tests again I had an appointment with EI. They were coming to our house with a team of different therapist, all with different specialties. They were going to evaluate Olivia to see if she was delayed in her development in any way. After a few hours with us their team let us know where they saw delays in our daughter, and how far behind she was. They also gave us a number of different resources for family support, medical help, financial help, and the therapies Olivia would need to try and get her up to age appropriate responses. They gave us websites to research all kinds of hearing related topics. They explained the process like no one else had. And most importantly they asked if we had gotten a second opinion from anyone on Olivia's hearing.

I started kicking myself at that moment. Why the heck hadn't we thought of a second opinion? After all the issues we had had with the people we were using, and how bad we felt with the idea of not doing anything else for Olivia because her good ear was good enough. Had we done this to our child? Were we to blame for her delays? Why didn't anyone ever tell us about EI before her first birthday? It has taken me years to get over this. In fact on some days I am not quite sure I am totally over it, but mostly I am. They recommended a local hospital. I was on the phone with our insurance and then the hospital within an hour of the EI team leaving our house. We never went back to the audiologist or the ENT we were using. Instead we started working with the staff at the local hospital and got a lot more information and resources for our daughter.

I guess from all of this we learned a couple of very important lessons. Trust your gut. If it doesn't sound right to you, or sit right with you, found out why. Don't just take one "expert's" opinion. Get a second or third opinion if you need it. You are not alone. Some of the resources from EI put us in touch with other parents going through the same thing. It is not easy to be a hearing parent trying to figure out how to raise and care for a deaf or hard of hearing child. But you don't have to face it alone. You can get in touch with other experts: the parents who have traveled this road before you. They may make different choices than you will, but they have walked in your shoes. They understand how it feels when you think no one else understands what you are going through. They can and will help you along the way.

Olivia started Hearing Therapy once a week, then Speech Therapy as well. Later it was decided she would also benefit from Occupational Therapy. Each one helped our little girl get stronger, and catch up to what an age appropriate child could do. I signed up for every website on hearing loss I could find. I read everything I could get my hands on. One day there was an email about Mom's Night Inn, for mothers of kids who were deaf or hard of hearing. I didn't know anyone, and was a little worried about going, but I decided to step out of my comfort zone and go anyway. I did get my own room. I guess I could only go so far out of my comfort zone. I even brought a book, my laptop, a movie on DVD to play on the laptop and a blanket I was trying to crochet. So I had all of my own things to do in case it didn't work out.

Well after getting set up in my hotel room, and going over the agenda I went down for my first session, but still brought my crochet bag with me. I think it was like my armor. If I was not comfortable talking to people I didn't know I could just sit and crochet or it could have been something to talk about with someone new. I am not sure which way I thought it was going to work out. I did crochet a bit during the breaks, but I have to say they had the Mom's Night so well planned that I did meet some very nice women. We shared our stories, we listened to a great guest speaker, we had dinner, and got a chance to just relax. There were activities and things to keep us busy, like manicures and massages. But the best part of the weekend was all the great information that was shared.

There was information in our gift bags on things like Parent's Institute, and guest speakers who talked about colleges for deaf students, all things I didn't know. But the best information I got was the different stories from the Mom's with kids that were older than mine. They very kindly shared their tales of how they dealt with different issues that came up in their family; like when your child doesn't want to keep their hearing aids in, or when some doctor tells you what you have to do for your child, or even when family and friends don't understand that your child is pretty much like any other child. It was great. I have gone back again, and I don't think I would miss one in the future if I could help it.

I took all of that information from Mom's Night Inn and went over it my husband. We did go to the Parent's Institute that June. It was one week for us to go down as a family and learn more about hearing loss, how to read an audiogram, learn some things about Deaf life and experiences, take sign language classes, and even have time to relax and play as a family. My husband was not sure if he should take off work and if we should all go, but afterwards he did say it was the best thing we could have done for our family. It was a great opportunity to get our child evaluated and to meet other families that were going through the same things we were. All the families have a deaf or hard of hearing child that is five or younger. They were all learning as they went along too. We had the opportunity to meet with a number of different experts on children with hearing loss. I am not sure what was the most valuable, but the whole experience really helped us to navigate this journey that we are on.

One thing from that week that stuck with me was finding out that our child would be evaluated by a psychologist. I didn't really understand why, and was a bit afraid of this. But I have to say it went very well. In fact when we met with him, after he had evaluated our daughter, he told us she was ahead of her age development in socializing. Olivia was 21 months old, was developmentally at 34 – 36 months old. This was the first time anyone had ever told us Olivia was ahead in any area. In fact he went on to tell us a few more areas where she was at or above her age level in development. Sure there were areas where she was behind, but we knew that. This information about the positive was new for us. I guess everyone had been so focused on the negatives, or the challenges--that they never thought to tell us the positives. I believe this is just as important as the challenges. We have to celebrate what our kids can do. This information was really a gift that I could not put a price on.

We also learned about our state's Deaf Mentor program from another mother at the Institute and decided to request one. Having a Deaf Mentor brought a great role model into our home and we were able to ask all kinds of questions about growing up and daily life. She helped our family learn ASL and introduced us to Deaf Culture. We enjoyed watching Olivia turn our Deaf Mentor's head from side to side to see her hearing aids and see the joy she had of sharing this common bond.

Olivia just started preschool and she currently has no delays—she is at or above age development in every area. She recently experienced more hearing loss so our path has once again turned in a new direction.

When you are pregnant you dream about the baby that is on the way. Most parents dream of the "perfect" baby. That usually involves counting ten fingers and ten toes. At first with Olivia she seemed to meet this definition, and yet at the same time she didn't. It has taken a lot of ups and downs along the way. But we have learned a lot more about that picture. Thanks to Olivia, we have learned that there are many different definitions of the word perfect, and that Olivia really is perfect.

Never underestimate what deaf and hard of hearing kids can accomplish, never put limits on them, and encourage them to follow their dreams.

~ Beth Donofrio

Chapter 3
Married to the Method

Each day of our lives we make deposits in the memory banks of our children.

~ Charles R. Swindoll

I've always been perplexed at how parents of newly diagnosed babies are expected to examine all the choices related to communication methods and then these parents are expected to "pick one." There's an expectation that if you simply pick a method and stick with it, your child will grow up to successfully communicate with that method. And if your child didn't succeed with the chosen method, then sakes alive, you didn't do your job as a parent to make that happen. Tsk, tsk.

If you're a lucky parent, you'll have contact with a parent, professional or deaf/hard of hearing adult who can guide you through this process without bias.

And what does it mean, this term "without bias?" In a nutshell, it means that the person giving support does it in a way that doesn't have an agenda behind it or the intention of steering you down a certain path. For this, I give a huge credit to Hands & Voices You can read more about support without bias on their website: www.handsandvoices.org.

After David's diagnosis, we were bombarded with advice from well-meaning friends, relatives, professionals and other parents. Some were convinced their communication mode/method was the Holy Grail for deaf and hard of hearing children and they were quick to let me know. I've met folks passionate about every mode or methodology. To say they're passionate would be an understatement for some. Passion is a great thing when shared without coercion. Passion becomes a bad thing when you toss in judgment, coercion, railroading and superiority, all of which I've experienced on this journey. The hardest part for me as a parent was to deal with folks who were so "married to the method" they wanted me to join in on the marriage too.

And sometimes, as a parent, you can't see any of it coming at you.

I had well-meaning friends tell me their opinions about what I should be doing with my kids and some would become upset with my decisions. Well-meaning professionals tossed in their educated guesses as well. There were some days I doubted my path with my kids. There were other days I felt confident and comfortable.

Janet Des Georges, Executive Director of Hands & Voices said something profound at a conference. Whenever there is doubt, she looks to her child as the "true North." What is your baby/child telling you? What do you know to be true about your baby/child—that truth will guide you in all of your decisions.

When it comes to raising deaf and hard of hearing children, we often talk about choices. When parents receive a diagnosis, they're sometimes introduced to an array of communication choices. Then they go home and study them and decide which one/s they're going to use to communicate with their child.

In theory, it all sounds like a nice process. Peruse your choices, pick one and apply it to your child. There's often a message of, "Well, if you do A, B, and C, you'll produce E. F, and G within the child. It's not that simple. In reality, there's a smorgasbord of other things to consider when raising a deaf or hard of hearing child. What works for one may not be right for another. Take a look at the many things that have an influence on the outcome (source: Hands & Voices):

Cause of hearing loss, degree, age of onset
Age of child
Educational options
Social Isolation
Technology
Family dynamics
Resources
Peers
...and more...

You can have two people with very similar audiograms, but very different abilities to process and understand the sound going in their heads.

But there is one thing that is constant: the human need for love and connection. We want to be able to communicate the thoughts in our head and heart to another human being and we want to be understood. We want to be able to understand others. That's what we need to focus on as parents—how do we do that to the deepest possible level? What does our child need for us to accomplish that?

Sometimes the forceful, passionate opinions of others can be difficult to deal with, especially if you're in a position where you're trying to consider different choices and perhaps not quite sure what direction you want to go in. Everything is all new, emotions are raw, and the amount of information is overwhelming.

> **I stand on this claim: I should not design a small language, and I should not design a large one. I need to design a language that can grow. I need to plan ways in which it might grow—but I need, too, to leave some choices so that other persons can make those choices at a later time.**
>
> ~Guy Steel

Over the years, I've learned that opinions are just that: opinions. You can ask ten different people/professionals for their opinion and you'll come up with ten different perspectives.

When I first began supporting families, I was not familiar with all of the communication choices out there. So I set out to learn everything I could. And over the years, I've had the wonderful opportunity to meet families from all walks of life using all of the possible modes and methods out there. My kids have been really fortunate to hang with kids who speak, cue, sign, combine, you-name-it.

I have found for every "communication success story" out there, there are others who may not have had similar outcomes.

I once asked a Chicago family how they came to their conclusion of what was right for their family and how they made the choices they did. "I didn't want to just tell my kid the sky is blue," said the father. "Not only did I want to tell him the sky was blue, I wanted to be able to explain to him in great detail precisely what made the sky blue, down to the scientific and the spiritual." The family went on to fight for this communication method for their son in the court system and ended up creating a private school as well.

If you're just starting out on the journey, sometimes it is wise not to make *any* decisions, but to sit back and use the time to gather information. Use the time to meet other families with children of all ages and backgrounds. Connect with as many different deaf and hard of hearing kids, teens and adults that you can.

It then boils down to this: you take everything you've learned, take what you know about your child, take in consideration what's in your heart… and make a decision.

Over time, you may make different choices. The path may twist and turn. Your child will grow older and weigh in on those decisions.

The bottom line becomes this: can you connect with your child on the deepest level possible? Can your child express his/her thoughts to the best of their ability?

I would encourage you to follow your instincts. You know your child more than anyone else. A wonderful doctor once told me that *I* am the expert on Henry, and that I should have a little more confidence in myself and not be afraid that I'm doing the wrong thing.

That was a valuable piece of information.

Of course you want to seek out opinions from experts, but you must also learn to think of yourself as an important piece of the "expert puzzle." Without you, the puzzle is incomplete.

Kristen
www.nosmallthing.wordpress.com

The following contribution is from Sally Skyer. I met Sally at the ALDACon, a conference for late-deaf adults.

This is what worked for Sally and her family; but keep in mind, it's not about the method, it's about building language bridge with your child by having fun, regardless of how.

Read...Sign...Talk...
And Have Fun Along the Way

~ Solange C. Skyer

As a born-deaf mom married to a late-deafened spouse, I was most concerned about making sure my hearing children would not experience any language or speech delays. Having firsthand experience with not speaking or able to read until I was five years old, I wanted to be sure my children would not face the same delay I experienced.

My husband and I bought several children's books including a collection of Mother Goose poems. We also collected books with accompanying sing/read along cassette tapes. I started reading/signing Mother Goose songs the first day we brought our daughter, Melissa, home from the hospital. I would prop her on her cradle and would sing Mother Goose songs and stories in varying cadence. I would sign with animated facial expressions making sure she had my full attention. If I was not reading or singing, I would talk/sign about what I was doing. I talked almost non-stop. I felt that constant exposure to speech/language and signing would set the foundation for developing strong spoken/expressive language. My husband would do the same…using his deep baritone voice; he would sing old familiar songs while rocking our daughter to sleep. Even if our speech was not perfect, we felt it was important for Melissa to hear our voices and connect with us through our language, our signs and facial expressions. We tried to incorporate fun by using play as an opportunity to talk/sign. We would watch "Sesame Street" and sing along. We would read books and use funny antics to reflect the story line. After our second child, Michael, joined us I continued with our play/reading time. Melissa started signing and using words when she was barely nine months old. By the time she turned one, she started using two word sentences. Her signing grew exponentially. By the time her brother, Michael, came along she would read/sing to him to sleep.

Melissa and Michael are now young adults. Both are voracious readers and are phenomenal communicators. They are proficient signers and are able to adapt communication with whomever they are interacting with. Both have straddled the deaf and hearing world comfortably. Both were taught to speech read from the time they were babies so that they would have adequate communication tools in the event they lose their hearing like their dad. Both have since lost their hearing and are adapting well.

In looking back, I am grateful for the emphasis on language development and am especially glad that we incorporated fun activities as part of language development. Our weekends and summers were filled with art activities, cooking lessons, dinner dialogues as well as interactions with hearing/deaf children and hearing/deaf adults. We made learning fun…We made our interaction educational.

The Communication Journey... For my Own Family

The communication journey was an interesting process with my children. David attended a program for deaf and hard of hearing kids from the time he was three until kindergarten. The teacher used simultaneous communication-- signing and speaking at the same time. He was comfortable signing and speaking or one without the other. Lauren, on the other hand, wanted nothing to do with signing in any way. She would constantly insist that she didn't need me to sign to her. Steven, with his quirky personality, was barely communicating.

Between birth to age five is the time period when we're told to cram as much exposure to language as possible. By age seven, we're told that if we don't maximize and optimize our child's development, then we've lost a window of opportunity for them to develop a full grasp of language and thought processing. This is for all kids in general. But when you've got a kid with a limited ability to hear and understand all that goes on around him, it becomes even more daunting for parents of deaf and hard of hearing kids to cram as much language development as possible into a few short years.

And consider this: the sense of hearing is fully developed at 20 weeks in utero. This means a developing infant with normal hearing gets exposed to the sounds in the environment long before they're born. A baby with a profound hearing loss is born already 20 weeks behind in terms of hearing stimulation. So we're playing catch up from the minute that the umbilical cord is cut.

Now back to cramming language development. I've met some families who take the task so seriously that it becomes a grind for the whole family. That's where play comes into... well... play! My kids' absolute favorite time of the day was bath time. For me, that time was teaching time, only my kids didn't really know it. That's where they learned to read. Yes, in the bathtub. The best thing I ever bought for my kids was a set of foam letters and numbers. The wet foam stuck to the bathroom walls. I started off by introducing one or two letters at a time when they were about eight months old. They quickly learned to identify letters just as they identified a dog or cat. Then I'd stick an "A" and "B" on the wall. They would learn those two letters. Then I'd toss the A and B with the letters all floating in the water. "Where's the A?" I would ask, and I'd fingerspell the "A." The kids would hunt in the water for the "A" and slap it on the tile wall. Off we'd go to hunt for "B" and so on.

As the kids became more familiar with the letters, I'd spell out "cat" and "dog" on the wall. "Cat starts with a 'C'" I'd explain. "Which word is 'cat'?" Then I'd take off the "t" and replace it with a "p." Oh look, the new word is "cap!" I'd grab the hubby's cap and show them.

Bath time was also ice cream time. There's no more perfect place for popsicles and little chubby hands than in a bath tub. So what if it drips down-- the bath water is the perfect diluter. They learned their colors with popsicles. "Do you want a purple or red one?" M & M's were another great color-and-counting tool.

What can I say--I raised my kids on junk food. But hey, they learned their colors! And ABCs!

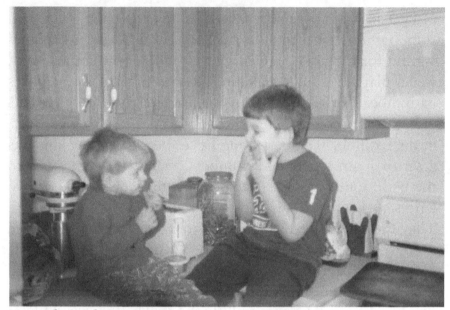

David teaching Steven

I also did a lot of activities in the kitchen with the kids. From the time they were toddlers, I taught them math with whatever we were baking or cooking at the time. "Can you hand me two eggs?" The back of the brownie box was perfect for those early math skills as it was easy to spot the graphic with two eggs. We'd hunt for the ¼ line on the measuring cup and fill it with oil. As they got older, I'd up the challenge. "If I fill this to the ¼ line, how much more would I need to fill it to reach one cup?" Needless to say, we ate a lot of brownies.

Once I knew my kids' skills were solid in one area, I'd play the "Mommy's wrong" game. If we were playing a spelling game, I would spell a word wrong (one that I knew they would know) and they took great delight in correcting Mommy's mistakes. Or I'd add something up wrong or identify the wrong color, etc. This was a great exercise to play, because I could also tell if they were paying attention and getting full access to our communication... or not.

When I look back to my early years, I learned this teaching skill from my father. He dropped out of school in 8th grade to work on a farm, but he was a smart man. Even after double shifts at the office, he would tell me a story at bedtime. He taught me to spell "encyclopedia" at the age of three. I grew up reading from those very books after he bought the entire Encyclopedia Britannica set.

My daughter gave me a new appreciation for understanding communication in all its forms. I used to sit with my hands in my lap and only listen to words. Now I watch people, read more body language, and use more than I ever have before... and I would have never learned that without a firsthand experience with a child who would reach up to my cheeks and turn my face to make sure I was listening to her. (Not looking means not listening, right?)

~ Sara Kennedy

I had a conversation with Carrie Balian, the Director of the Illinois Guide By Your Side program and mother to 12-year-old Jack. In the middle of their journey with Jack, their path took twists and turns they could not have imagined in the beginning. "It's been a great journey," said Carrie. "I've learned when you make a decision, it's not a decision you're stuck with forever. You can do a 360--or whatever you want to call it—the decisions are not set in stone. A good decision, a bad decision, it's all part of the process. I've learned to keep an open mind. You don't have to commit to one thing forever-- and it will be okay."

The one lesson Carrie learned was to always get a second and even a third opinion when exploring the decisions. "It never really occurred to me to get other opinions in the beginning," she said. "Think about it, when you buy a car, you do your research, you shop around, you visit different dealers, and you test-drive the cars. As a parent, getting other opinions and input will help you come to terms with the decisions you make and what you choose to do."

And one more thing, Carrie says. "Make sure you make time to enjoy the journey. In the beginning, I was so overwhelmed going from one appointment to the next, and always trying to please the therapists. Our play became too much like therapy all the time. They're only little for a short time—take the time to enjoy them and appreciate them. It's not always about hearing loss. Don't get so wrapped up in the diagnosis, or the therapy that you miss all the milestones-- or that you forget to enjoy your kid."

When David was diagnosed, my husband and I were already signing to him and he had developed speech at that point. So we continued to develop both his signing and speaking skills. The hubby and I had deaf, hard of hearing and hearing friends and we just wanted the kids to be able to interact with everyone around us.

There were two things that scared me as a parent of a deaf kid: the 4th grade reading levels which kept turning up in my research and the "use it or lose it" philosophy about amplifying residual hearing in kids. Yeah, at the time, those were the two things I stressed over. As a kid growing up, I loved to read, and the written word provided me access to the parts of the auditory world which I could not access. The one thing the hubby and I did every night was to read before bedtime. We had board books in every nook and cranny of the house. Soon, I discovered I didn't have to worry about the reading issue—David loved to read and he looked forward to digging into books.

But the one thing we battled over was keeping the hearing aids in. Shortly after David received his first hearing aid, it went missing. We were outside in the backyard, sitting with the neighbors and the kids were running around. It was late in the evening and I noticed that a hearing aid was missing from David's ear. So we assembled a team and strolled up and down the back yard, looking for the missing hearing aid.

"Where is your hearing aid?" I asked the toddling David. He just shrugged. Nighttime came, and we continued to march up and down the backyard with flashlights. The search continued the next day, until we finally gave up. The hearing aid was nowhere to be found.

Six months later, it finally turned up: at the bottom of a wicker toy basket.

The hearing aid battle continued, with the stubborn toddler winning most of the rounds. I finally hit on a solution: if the kiddo wanted to watch TV or a video, then the hearing aids had to stay in. As soon as a hand reached to pluck it out, the TV went off. They quickly learned to comply if they wanted to watch their favorite cartoon or the 200th replay of a Pokemon video. As they became older, wearing the hearing aids became a non-issue, as they grew to appreciate the sounds they could hear with them on. We still had to play hunt-for-the-hearing aids every now and then when someone would absent-mindedly forget where they took off their aids. We've lost several hearing aids over the years.

As a parent, when my kids were very young, I quickly learned to give my kids choices that I could live with. "Do you want to wear the red shirt or the yellow shirt today? The blue jeans or the sweat pants?" If a kid wanted to battle for something else, like wearing shorts in the dead of winter, I weighed everything with relevance. Did the battle really matter? What were the consequences? Would the decision matter one hour, one month, one year later-- or heck, would it scar the kid for life? This stuff didn't just apply to clothes, it applied to everything. I learned to choose my battles carefully.

I am a deaf father of two boys, one deaf and one hearing. My experience growing up has taught me the importance of having excellent reading skills and for deaf and hard of hearing people it is a critical skill to build for your success and survival in the 'hearing world'. It is sometimes hard to explain this importance to your kids and have them realize its value at an early age. As a result, they'll just procrastinate with reading or complain that it's too hard and boring. I certainly remember that was how it started for me. Fortunately, I was able to break through and that was with comic books!

Although comic books are loaded with tons of drawings and you'd think that's no proper way to learn how to read. Indeed, the many facial expressions, body language and actions that I tried to 'read' had unconsciously encouraged me to start reading the words in the spoken bubbles. I have fond childhood memories of those tall stacks of Archie and G.I Joe comic book series. Naturally, the comic books were more fun and seemed easier to read. The more I read of them, the better my reading skills became. I soon graduated to the popular MAD magazines then on to newspapers, novels and print magazines. Should your children have difficulties with reading, encourage them to do additional reading on the side with comic books. The more reading that's done; of any kind, the easier it gets.

~ Steve Murbach, father to Kyle, National Merit Scholar

Chapter 4
Twists and Turns on the Journey

The road of life twists and turns and no two directions are ever the same. Yet our lessons come from the journey, not the destination.

~ Don Williams

Sometimes on the course of the journey of raising deaf and hard of hearing kids, the path changes in ways we can't imagine. As our kids get older, they begin to weigh in on our decisions and make decisions of their own. Sometimes their decisions go against everything we've known on the journey. They may run off the path towards a gnarly forest when we want to keep them in freshly-mowed field where we can watch over them.

At Hands & Voices, we have a saying that we share with parents: "Nothing is set in stone." You can always change something. The whole parenting gig is a learning process and frankly, we don't stop learning until we take our final breath.

When Lauren was young, she refused to have anything to do with American Sign Language. As she became older, her views began to soften and she started picking up the language. When she came home from a camp out of state, she decided she would no longer wear her hearing aids. We supported her decision. A few weeks later, the hearing aids were parked back in her ears. Soon after that, she joined a deaf drama group and began performing songs in ASL.

We enrolled her in a high school with 80 other deaf kids and she began using an interpreter. Two years later, she transferred to our local high school and chose not to use an interpreter.

Twists and turns, indeed.

Over the summer, I talked to two moms who both started off on similar paths with their kids and they encountered different paths along the way.

Trisha Thelen's Parenting Journey:

When Marina was 13-months-old, she stopped talking. At her 15-month checkup, I mentioned this to the pediatrician and he first thought it was fluid in her ears. Tests later showed she was profoundly deaf. We were told hearing aids wouldn't work for her, but we decided to go ahead and try them anyway. The hearing aids worked well and Marina wanted to use them every day. When she was four, we began to notice her hearing declining. Some days she could hear well, other days she could hear nothing. She was diagnosed with Pendred Syndrome, which also affects the thyroid and kidneys.

We were cautioned to keep her safe from blows to the head or she could lose more hearing. When she was seven, Marina crashed into a tree while sledding. She was wearing a helmet. She lost the rest of her hearing that she could hear with hearing aids.

That's when our journey with cochlear implants began. She received her first one on the right ear. Two years later, the skin became raw at the site of the magnet so Marina took off the implant for six months. We opted for a second implant on her other ear. Meanwhile, we continued to have problems with the right. The implant began malfunctioning and she experienced shocks from it. The surgeons replaced the implant with a new one. When she was thirteen, the site became infected and the nerves had grown around the implant. We went back and forth on the idea of implanting again with Marina's input, and she decided to have it implanted again.

Throughout the ordeal, Marina experienced pain from the nerves surrounding the implant. Some days she would go to school in a lot of pain. The doctor put her on steroids, but it didn't help. Last January, we had the implant removed completely. She had a total of six surgeries by this point. The surgeon suggested cutting the nerve to relieve the pain.

It was up to Marina to decide if she wanted to try another implant or just cut the nerve and be done with that ear. We let her decide herself, as we don't know what it's like from her perspective and we don't know what it's like to be her. She decided to go for another implant since she was having the surgery anyway. The surgeon put the implant in a new location and cut the nerve which was causing her pain. She has no more pain and the new implant works fine. She's gone through a lot, yet she's well-adjusted.

At the beginning of our journey, the professional who did the ABR ended up changing out the machine after she first tested Marina. "I've never seen a baby this deaf," she said. They discovered Marina didn't have balance function on one side. They predicted she wouldn't be able to walk or talk. A doctor told us if we didn't teach Marina to speak she would only get a job at Burger King. We had professionals telling us things and giving advice that turned out to be wrong—that was the biggest challenge. I got mad. This only motivated me to raise Marina as a well-rounded person. She speaks. She signs. She graduated with honors, went to Italy by herself over the summer and she's now in college. She has a lot of hearing friends and deaf/hard of hearing friends. We don't know what it's like to be deaf, we felt Marina needed to be around others who are deaf and hard of hearing to connect and understand each other.

I would never tell another parent what to do--you have to do what's best for your child. It was a challenge not to get upset with others who thought they knew what was best for us. What we did worked for us. I don't have any regrets and I wouldn't change anything. If we changed it, she would be a different person today.

To a parent new on the journey, my advice is simple: follow your heart and your instincts. Go with your gut. Talk with other parents and learn from them. If you're not comfortable with a professional find a new one. You need professionals on your journey every step of the way, including deaf and hard of hearing people. I think you have to sometimes stand your ground and fight for what you want.

In the end it's all worth it.

Debbie Bernabei's Parenting Journey:

"The journey has changed directions so many times," said Debbie Bernabei. Debbie is the mom of Kurt, a sandy-haired teen who loves hockey. "We started out with hearing aids with Kurt and he received some benefit from them, we were seeing some results in the sound booth. I struggled with the decision of whether or not to get an implant, but I didn't want to change Kurt. He was fine just the way he was. I wanted to change myself to fit him. I didn't want him to feel broken-- that was my big thing. I didn't want him to feel that he needed to be fixed."

So Debbie dove into interpreting classes and learned American Sign Language. Her husband and extended family spent hours soaking up the language.

When Kurt was nine, he asked about getting a cochlear implant. Several of his friends had implants and he wanted to hear more than what he could with his hearing aids. So after some research and information gathering, we went ahead with the surgery.

For two years, things hummed along. In sixth grade, things began to unravel. The itinerant teacher discovered that Kurt was taking off his implant and putting it in his pocket. She insisted that he had to wear it in school. But little did we know, Kurt was popping out the battery case so that it was off. Everything came pouring out during a visit to the audiologist in the fall that year. "It's too much stress," he said. "I'm trying to focus on the interpreter in class and the sound is bothering me." We had a long talk about the implant and from that point on, he never wore it again.

Looking back, I could see the signs of stress here and there. As soon as he would arrive home after school, he would take the implant off. During the summer, I would have to fight with him to keep it on.

From the time he was two, we had faced that decision whether or not to get an implant. He was getting some benefit from hearing aids and deep down, I didn't want to change Kurt. I wanted to change myself to fit him. I didn't want him to feel as if he was broken and needed to be "fixed" by giving him an implant. By the time he expressed interest in the implant, we thought it might help him sound out words better. But it also made me question my choices along the journey-- was I wrong before? You can't wait for a child to decide-- parents have to make the decisions.

From the time he was little, Kurt always accepted himself. He's proud to be deaf. He doesn't hide his signing, nor does he try to fit into the hearing world. He has hearing friends but he knows he doesn't have conversations with them the same way as he does with his deaf friends. We set up a Sign Club at school and 35 kids signed up. Kurt stays after school and teaches them along with his interpreter.

Yes, I've looked back and questioned my choices along the journey. But I've learned as a parent, you have to make decisions that are right for NOW. Sometimes the path will change along the journey.

So, what I am learning and realizing is that this journey is quite a rollercoaster ride or maybe a bit like surfing: you work hard, you work through the uncertain times and the times when you struggle and don't know what to do...you find the knowledge and find the strength and skills to carry on and do what needs to be done...and then when these precious developments happen, the reward is like some sort of natural drug--a blissful state of joy that completely consumes you and fills your heart and makes it bounce.

~ Gina Watt, mom of Sara

Chapter 5
The Macaroni and Cheese Story

Run your fingers through my soul. For once, just once, feel exactly what I feel, believe what I believe, perceive as I perceive, look, experience, examine, and for once; just once, understand.

~ Unknown

I was visiting a family with a two-and-a-half-year-old hard of hearing son—providing mentoring services as part of weekly early intervention services. In the middle of a question and answer session, the mom shared an experience which puzzled her. Earlier in the week, her son went into the pantry and came out with a box of macaroni and cheese. He pointed to the picture of the creamy bowl of macaroni and cheese and tapped it several times.

"You want some macaroni and cheese?" she asked.

"Yes!" He nodded excitedly as she opened the box. He tried to grab the box from her.

"No, wait, Stephen," she said. "I have to cook it."

He stamped his feet, tried to grab the box again with an impatient look on his face. She tried to explain the cooking process, but he wanted to have nothing of it. He wanted the macaroni and cheese that was displayed on the box.

The mom looked at me with a quizzical look on her face. "I don't understand this," she said. "I never had to explain this to my older girls. They knew the macaroni and cheese from the box had to be cooked."

"Ok," I said. "Let's look at how it's different for your son compared to your hearing daughters. Let's say that the girls are playing in the next room. You call out to them, 'Want some macaroni and cheese?' and they yell back, 'Yes!' They hear you walk over to the pantry and take out the box. They probably hear the rattle of the hard macaroni as it jiggles around in the box. You open another cabinet, grab a pot and then walk over to the sink. They hear the clang of the pot in the sink and the rush of the water as it fills up the pot. You turn off the water and then walk over to the stove. The pot clatters on the top of the stove and then there's the click as you turn the gas on."

All the while the hearing kids are playing in the next room, there are a bunch of auditory sounds that may seem like they don't convey much information, but the pieces gather in their brain and together, they tell the whole story. Deaf and hard of hearing kids may miss this information completely or they may only gather bits and pieces of it.

"Then the kids hear the rip as the box top is sheared off and the hard noodles hit the bubbling water." I continued. "They hear the drawer open as you grab a spoon and then they hear metal upon metal as the noodles are stirred. Right after you turn off the stove, there's the sound of the colander settling in the sink. The noodles dribble down into the colander while the water splashes through the holes."

(And perhaps the kids are privy to a few sharp words as you accidentally hit the hot pot with your bare knuckles.)

"The fridge door opens and you mutter to yourself, 'Where did I put the last stick of butter?' The cheese package gets ripped open, the milk hits the pan and everything gets mixed together. There's the clatter of the bowls and spoons and finally, the masterpiece is set on the table. 'Come and get your macaroni and cheese!' you holler to the girls. They walk into the kitchen and dig into the steaming noodles."

The mom sat there for a minute, completely stunned.

"Wow, I never realized how significant the insignificant sounds of the day could be," she said.

I tell this story to every parent that I mentor. You see, deaf and hard of hearing kids miss out on tons of audiological information during the day. If we don't find a way to fill in those blanks, then the child becomes language deprived and begins to fall behind their peers.

I encourage parents to become the ears for their kids, filling in the auditory information that they may not have access to. For example, when a parent arrives home from work, kids with normal hearing can hear the car drive up and the garage door opening. For deaf and some hard of hearing kids, the parent just suddenly appears out of nowhere. There are no pieces to fill in the auditory puzzle.

Another thing, when the phone rings and you start talking, does your deaf/hard of hearing kid have access to your conversation?

Think about it, kids with normal hearing have access to your phone conversations, however one-sided they may be. What does your deaf and hard of hearing kid access? That's something you have to examine and determine how you can provide that access to your child. You may think that a simple phone call is meaningless, but every little piece of information is significant. The hearing kid gets to know how many times a day Grandma calls. The hearing kid gets to hear Mom saying "I love you" at the end of a conversation when Dad calls in during his lunch break (and the kid concludes that they've made up after the argument he heard that morning). The hearing kid gets to hear his sister arguing with her best friend (and that explains why the friend isn't coming over for the last several days...).

You get the gist. Deaf and hard of hearing kids may have little or no access to the conversations that flow around them throughout the day. As a parent, you will have to get really creative on making sure you can fill in the auditory information gaps for your kid. And as a parent, you have to make sure you're not stepping in every single time and becoming the "interpreter" for your child. Sometimes that's a tough dance. As parents, you want your kid to access everything. But there will be times when you will have to step back and let your kid handle their own communication access.

One time, I met a new parent at a local McDonalds for a play date. David wanted to get an ice cream cone, so I gave him the money and he trotted off to the front counter. He was seven at the time. The other mom looked at me in amazement. She had always ordered for her deaf child, even from the menu in restaurants. It was time for her to start letting go, and let her child communicate directly.

Build those communication bridges early. Let your kid make mistakes. Let them struggle to connect with others. Let others get over their own struggles to communicate back with your kid.

And become innovative with the way everyone communicates. Do whatever it takes.

Take time to get to know your baby/child. Take time to be a family. The world is all yours-- and there are many choices out there for parents to explore. No one road is right for every child and family.

~ Karen Hopkins

Raising Scott

~ Anita Jones

I was in the kitchen dropping pots and pans when I noticed my seven-month-old son didn't respond to the sound. At his next checkup, I expressed my concerns to the doctor. He picked up a cowbell and told me to watch Scott's face. Well Scott didn't respond to the sounds. Two days later, Scott had an ABR test which confirmed our suspicions. My husband and I just sat there in silence, taking it all in. We shed some tears and we were at a loss as to what to do. We started probing for the "why" this happened—asking my OB questions and trying to get answers. We scoured the Internet for as much information as we could find. We quickly came to a conclusion: it was not important to dwell on the "why;" it was more important to pour language in him.

Within two weeks, we had early intervention services set up. While my husband was on a business trip, he visited Gallaudet and the AG Bell headquarters. We explored all the communication options and read everything we could. We looked at all kinds of schools across the country. We talked to parents, families and counselors all over. It was a big learning process for us.

In the morning, Scott would attend the state school for the deaf and in the afternoon he attended the gifted program at the local school. In middle school, he attended the local school where he was the only deaf kid. By high school, he chose to go to a high school with a deaf program. He graduated 23 out of his class of 500+ students.

Communicating with Scott wasn't difficult, it just took more time and effort. I speak fast, plus I tend to multi-task, so I had to train myself to make changes—to make sure I was making eye contact and shortening the distance between us. I was always checking to make sure we were on the same wavelength with what was being said as well as the emotions involved. In the car, I tilted the mirror and I would catch his eyes; and I made sure he could see my lips and hands move.

In every social situation, I took that as an opportunity to teach others how to include Scott and communicate with him. He was also missing out on incidental hearing—a door would close or the phone would ring—I made sure to communicate those things to him.

It was challenging to make sure everything was getting into his head. If he rolled his eyes at me, I was always asking myself if that was normal or if it was because I didn't make sense to him. I was never 100% sure what I said got through to him, but then again, every parent of a teenager worries about that.

Chapter 6
Every Child is a Gift

My father gave me the greatest gift anyone could give another person, he believed in me.

~ Jim Valvano

Every child is a gift. This is something I truly believe. A kid who has racked up a number of disabilities and conditions from his genetic pool has something to give to the world. The key is to find that gift... and show it to the world.

There's a story that always stands out in my mind when I talk with families with kids who have multiple disabilities. It's the story of Dick and Rick Hoyt. You might have heard of them. Or maybe not. But the story is a great one. Rick was born in 1962 with the umbilical cord wrapped around his neck. The lack of oxygen resulted in cerebral palsy and Rick was not able to speak. But through the use of technology, Rick communicated. One day, in 1977, Rick told his father that he wanted to participate in a five-mile run. Dick had no running experience, but he pushed Rick's wheelchair and they finished next to last.

Fast forward today-- the father/son duo has competed in over 1,000 races, including several Ironman triathlons. In running events, Dick pushed Rick's wheelchair. In biking events, Rick rode on the front of the bike. In swimming events, Dick swam with Rick strapped to a floating raft. The two of them have inspired folks from all over. When one of my friends ran his first triathlon, he kept an image of Dick and Rick in his mind when he wanted to give up. If a father could do an Ironman running, swimming and biking with his son, then my friend had no excuse not to push himself along every step of the way. Can you see the gift?

But the point I want to share with this story is that Rick had a desire to experience running a 5K along with his peers. At first glance, one might have looked at Rick in the wheelchair and responded to that desire by saying, "Impossible." or "The race is meant to be run and you can't run or move, how will you do it?" The world would have missed the gift from this duo if they had thought in terms of limitations.

And this is what we have to do with our kids—see the possibilities. Focus on what they can do. Focus on their gifts, skills and abilities. And just so I can emphasize this a bit further, there's a great quote from W. Mitchell, a guy who was burned in a car accident and then later paralyzed in a plane crash:

"Before I was paralyzed there were 10,000 things I could do. Now there are 9,000. I can either dwell on the 1,000 I've lost or focus on the 9,000 I have left."

Now let me introduce you to Heidi Zimmer. As a kid, she loved to climb things. One day, she decided to climb to the roof of their 1950's bungalow. She was two years old.

That was the start of her climbing career.

Today, she's aiming to be the first deaf person to reach all seven of the world's highest summits. She's climbed three of them so far. She was the first deaf woman to climb Mt. Denali and the first deaf person to climb Mt. Kilimanjaro and Mt. Elbrus.

"In the 1980's, I read a book called 'What Color is Your Parachute,'" said Heidi. There was a sentence in there that said, 'You're disabled, so what?' We tend to buy in to what society tells us, and the message is often one of pity or a victim attitude. When I first started climbing, people would often tell me the reasons why I couldn't do this or that. "You can't climb a mountain because you're a woman." What kind of rule is that? That's society's view of women. It's more important to listen to what's in your heart to guide your path in life."

Oh by the way, did I tell you… Heidi is deaf blind.

I've worked in early intervention with families for many years. And before I got into early intervention, I worked at a Center for Independent Living where my co-workers and consumers were all people with disabilities. We often encountered people in the community who could not see past our disabilities. All they could see were limitations. All they could see were the dollar signs of access. Jo Waldron of Bender Consultants often says, "Attitude is the worst barrier of all."

And what we need is a paradigm shift.

A paradigm shift is a simple concept-- it's a shift in thinking, a revolution, a metamorphosis. Thomas Kuhn calls it a shift of one world view to another. Lee Woodruff, in her book, Perfectly Imperfect, describes her own paradigm shift throughout her chapter, A Different Ability:

"Your daughter is deaf," the doctor said, and it seems to echo across the crowded London Clinic. It was such a final word, so frightening. After that first failed test in the pediatrician's office, we'd been through weeks of medical rigors to rule out unimaginable conditions and diseases that could be related to deafness. We'd endured months of worry, stemming from that first moment when eight-month-old Nora didn't hear the little silvery bell during what was supposed to be a routine checkup. And now, living in London, and the test were finally conclusive. Deaf was the word he used.

He said it in such a matter-of-fact, medical manner, as if it were just another day on the job and not my own baby daughter's life at hand. My first thought when he uttered those words was "Who will ever ask a little deaf girl to the prom?"

The chapter is a wonderful one, as Lee unfolds the experience of getting to know her daughter. As the years go on, the paradigm shifts for her. Her pink hearing aids become just another part of her child, mixed in with all the budding talents emerging from within.

"Now when I think back to those early days of discovery in London, I am somewhat amused to recall my initial despair," Lee writes. "It was a lesson I have been shown more times than I could have imagined when I stood as a young bride, about to take the stage of the rest of my life as a woman, wife and, ultimately, mother. Back then, I hadn't really understood the overarching capacity people have to adapt, to be patient, and to recover. I hadn't factored in the resilience of the human spirit, the very real healing powers of time passing, the grace and perspective we find in moments of repose, and the ability of the soul to regenerate.

"In those long-ago days I saw a daughter with a disability. Now I see a beautiful, engaging person with a different ability, one that has blessed her with extra gifts and special perceptions."

How beautiful is that… the gift of a different ability.

Making the decision to have a child is momentous. It is to decide forever to have your heart go walking around outside your body.

~ Elizabeth Stone

What I Learned From My Hard of Hearing Daughter

~ Julie Vassilatos

What have I learned from my hard-of-hearing daughter? All sorts of things she never meant to teach.

First. Things are often not what I thought they would be, or how I thought they should be. And once I set aside my preconceptions, this paves the way for understanding. For instance, my hearing-aided daughter does not always want help hearing. In fact she sometimes would rather not hear at all. The refrain "I'm done hearing now," uttered as she pulls her aids out and hands them to me after a long noisy day at kindergarten, used to startle and puzzle me; now I'm used to it, and as a matter of fact, sometimes I'm done hearing, too, but there's not much I can do about it.

Second, a hard-of-hearing child very often uses vision to compensate for a lack of hearing. And so, my daughter is a keen observer, spotting the pale moon in the sky on a sunny afternoon, seeing a small grasshopper concealed in the grass, meticulously copying words she sees and pictures she likes as she learns to read and draw. She helps me attune my attention to visual detail.

And the third, I'm embarrassed to admit. Hearing loss has nothing in itself to do with lack of intelligence. I don't know. Maybe I was too close to the situation. Maybe she was just little and obstinate and I never noticed. But I was totally unaware of my daughter's intelligence until we had her evaluated for special services in public school. All I knew was, she just seemed never to understand anything, asking the same questions over and over, or looking at me blankly when I would make basic requests. (And this while I knew of her hearing loss.) Upon her evaluations it became clear that cognitively she was far ahead of where I thought. But because she was differently intelligent than her brother, and because she simply could not express herself clearly, and frequently not understand me, I had assumed she was a little dim, a little ditzy, or just plain not all there.

Now she is five, and enjoys math so much she sort of puzzles things out in her head for fun. "Mom," she called tonight from the table while I was fixing dinner. "Mom, three sixes is 18. Eight two's is also 18." Yes, you're right, I told her. Who told you that? "Nobody, mom, I just figured it out." I wonder, sometimes. If I hadn't had a staff of professionals—strangers both to me and my daughter— telling me that she was not lacking in intelligence, would I still be secretly believing that she had a diminished mental capacity because she has a diminished ability to hear? Would I not have finally understood that a lack of communication access is simply that? Would I not have realized that a small investment of extra patience, quiet listening, and focus on my daughter's dogged efforts at verbal clarity would reap huge dividends of understanding, respect, and learning? I don't know.

What I do know is that this tiny hard-of-hearing child living in our home presents us with little lessons, inadvertently, every day. If I heed them, I will be far the better for it.

Chapter 7
Killing Trees with All the IEP Paperwork

Education is not preparation for life; education is life itself.

~ John Dewey

The amount of paperwork with three kids in special education was enough to warrant an entire file drawer after a few years. I was no stranger to IEP meetings as I had advocated at a few of them during my first job. But it is one thing to advocate for someone else's child, and it's a whole other ballgame to sit through an IEP meeting as a parent. Sometimes you can't think straight when the emotions cloud your thoughts.

Speaking of emotions, this leads me to recommend "From Emotions to Advocacy," the special education survival guide written by Pam and Pete Wright. Visit www.wrightslaw.com for an amazing wealth of information that will prepare you well for your child's IEP meetings. "The Complete IEP Guide" by Lawrence Siegel is another book I recommend. Hands & Voices has an excellent book on advocating for your child in an educational setting: "Educational Advocacy."

Before you attend your first IEP, put together a few pages about your child and include some photos. This is a great way to introduce your kid to the team and share some personal information.

To prepare for your first IEP, there is an IEP Checklist as well as the "Pop Up IEP" with answers to common questions available on the Hands & Voices website:

http://www.handsandvoices.org/pdf/IEP_Checklist.pdf

I learned right away that having a perfect IEP is a myth—there will always be things that go awry or teachers who are unaware of what's on the IEP. Janet Des Georges and I teamed up and wrote *The Myth of the Perfect IEP: After the Paperwork is Finished.* One of the most crucial pieces of advice in that article is to find someone who can act as the MVP of your team:

> *Among the team that is assembled to deliver the services and supports for your child throughout the year, there is often an MVP -that professional who goes the extra mile, who supports you when you are advocating for your child, who you tend to call on when there is a problem. Whether that person is your child's general ed. Teacher, sign language interpreter, Teacher of the deaf/hard of hearing or a speech language pathologist, you can create and sustain a positive relationship throughout the year by communicating regularly, contacting them when there are things to be celebrated, and not just complaints to be delivered etc. and to be able to create strategies for effective communication access.*

> *If you can't think of one person on your child's IEP that you would consider an MVP, start thinking about who you could begin a positive relationship with in order to be able to collaborate with throughout the year, and be able to call upon for help when something falls through the cracks.*

I always tell parents they need to see themselves as the case manager for their child. The idea of acting as case managers on the IEP team may strike some parents as strange, because hey, aren't schools supposed to be doing that job? But here's something to think about, *parents* are the ones living daily with their child from the time they enter the family to the rest of their life. Parents are the one steady part of the IEP team that is always there.

The one tip I always share with parents is to keep all their paperwork in a binder. Being the disorganized mom I was—I was forever scrambling to find the latest IEP or audiograms for my kids.

~ Karen Putz

When the Team Doesn't Agree

My first encounter with opposition at an IEP meeting occurred during David's kindergarten year. The supervisor of the deaf education program had a strong opinion about moving David out of the self-contained classroom and placing him at our home district elementary school where he would be the only deaf kid. For Joe and I, our first reaction was an emphatic *no*. We wanted David to grow up with deaf and hard of hearing peers.

We were in a quandary though. David was extremely bright and he was producing work that was far above his grade level. The other children were either at grade level or below, so the teacher had to juggle her lessons to accommodate David in the classroom. It was becoming more and more apparent that his current placement was not meeting his needs, nor challenging his learning.

The more we thought about it and the more we explored our options (which is a joke-- more on that later), the more we realized putting David in our home elementary school was an option that we had to explore. There was another plus in our favor: the elementary school was brand new and all the students would be first-time students together. This gave us a chance to have David experience first grade along with the neighbor kids at the same time.

We signed the IEP paperwork with a bit of nervousness. One of the first things I did was to go into the new school and introduce myself to the principal. She listened intently as I described David and his education needs. I asked for her help in making the transition go smoothly with her staff and she agreed to partner with us to make the best of the placement. That initial meeting turned out to be the best thing-- as the principal attended nearly every IEP meeting after that for each of my three kids and she even advocated some situations for us.

David was assigned an interpreter who had deaf parents. She was personable and got along well with the other students. In fact, she was popular enough that the kids began to become fascinated with learning sign language and she set up a sign club after school. That first year, the entire school learned to sign the school song during assemblies. Every single year, the music teacher incorporated one signed song for every school musical performance. But this popularity proved to be difficult as well, for the students clamored for her attention and interaction. As a result, the interpreter would occasionally step out of the interpreting role and functioned as another teacher in the room. My husband and I weighed all the pros and cons of the experience and determined the pros far outweighed the cons. David's experience in our home district schools was a very positive one.

When Lauren and Steven arrived at the school, we still had some challenges here and there. Lauren did not use an interpreter, so we had to work harder with the staff to ensure that she had access in the classroom. Steven's first year proved to be an eye opener. I had long felt that I neglected my third child in the sense that he didn't get as much attention as the other two. There was one particular IEP meeting that I will never forget. Steven was in kindergarten and we were gathered around a table reviewing his test results. The itinerant teacher gave her report. The classroom teacher gave hers. The speech therapist gave hers.

The results were dismal.

"Steven is testing in the 15th percentile for language," the speech therapist explained. "We're concerned because he doesn't know some common vocabulary terms. He doesn't know what a penguin is."

I felt like a failure.

My five-year old-son could not identify a penguin.

My mind was quickly working up a defense. Hey--I never took the kid to the zoo to see the penguins! I never read him any books with penguins! I don't have any videos with penguins in them!

I knew I had dropped the ball with my kid, partly from the choices we made with his educational placement and partly because I (and the hubby too) wasn't devoting enough time in the day toward language development. But remember that smorgasboard of other things I talked about earlier which affects each family in different ways? We were also working with a child who was extremely shy-- so shy, that I came close to thinking perhaps he had Asperger's on the autism spectrum. He had trouble looking people in the eye when communicating. He insisted on macaroni and cheese for lunch for months and months at a time.

It was too late to change anything about the choices we made. But I could change my choices and actions from that point forward. So we dug in with the IEP team and came up with strategies to address his language learning. The following year, we had a much more positive IEP meeting and Steven was on track with his language development. In fact, he scored in the 80th percentile for language development. The IEP team was all smiles. I breathed a sigh of relief.

My kid finally knew what a penguin was.

Opposition is a natural part of life. Just as we develop our physical muscles through overcoming opposition - such as lifting weights - we develop our character muscles by overcoming challenges and adversity.

~ Stephen Covey

Yes, You Do Have Choices

One year, I was lamenting to Leeanne Seaver (Executive Director of Hands & Voices back then) about the limited "choices" which were available to my kids. I had to work within the school system. I had to deal with school boundaries while trying to get access to a mass of kids who could become peers. Some of the "professionals of the deaf" were sorely lacking in experience with working with and understanding the needs of deaf and hard of hearing students.

I whined.

Whined some more.

Then finally Leeanne said, "You do have options… you can move."

At first, I was indignant at her suggestion. I was supposed to pick up and *move* so I could get proper services for my kid? Are you kidding me?

The idea of choices is often a cold, hard reality for parents when they start out on the journey.

But Leeanne was right. We can choose to bloom where we're planted with our kids or we can pick up, move and plant seeds in a new place.

Blooming where you're planted…This can mean working like heck along with your team to make the changes you want to see in the system. It can mean finding innovative ways to create connections for your kids right where they are.

Jason Curry grew up in a small town. His parents wanted him to attend the local school with his brothers. For years, the other students attended sign classes during the school day. The students were eager to communicate with him and he grew up with many who became his close friends. When he graduated from elementary school, he finally learned the identity of the teacher who taught everyone to sign: his own mother. Today, Jason is the owner of sComm, a company that manufactures and distributes the UbiDuo, a communication device.

I've seen families go above and beyond to do whatever it takes for their kids. They'll drive hours and hours to get services or attend deaf and hard of hearing events.

One family had just moved into a new house when they received news that their deaf and hard of hearing co-op was redrawing the boundaries for some districts and pulling out of others. Their district was one of the pull-outs. The family quickly put a "for sale" sign out in front and moved into a district which could serve their child's needs. They had only been in their new house for a few months before they were filling up the moving truck once again.

Sometimes families feel powerless against strong advice from others. After a few years working with families, I began to notice a trend among Spanish-speaking families. Well-meaning professionals and medical personnel were advising them to focus only on English with their deaf and hard of hearing kids at home, even when the native language in the home was Spanish.

Hogwash.

Better advice: do whatever it takes to communicate with your kid. If Grandma only knows one language, let her teach it to your kid. Slap those little 3 X 5 notecards all over the house with the English word on it and whatever native language your family communicates in. Gesture, sign, cue, speak— whatever it takes. If the family speaks Klingon, then for crying out loud, include your kid on it.

I've worked with many families whose native language is Spanish and we simply incorporate it into our mentor activities with the kids. And boy did those families feed me well—we've had sessions centered around meals and language activities. I worked with one family who spoke Lithuanian in the home and today, the little first-grader is a pro in his family's native language and in English. In fact, the kid is above average in his language development skills at school.

Whatever it takes. Do it.

Advocating for your Deaf or Hard of Hearing Child

~ Andrea Marwah

Samantha is our miracle. It took three years and numerous rounds of infertility treatments to bring our miracle to us. We weren't aware of her hearing loss until she turned 2 years old. There were many other (much more debilitating) possibilities about Samantha's condition at that time. We were happy with the fact that it was hearing loss instead of other possibilities. We have faced obstacles and decisions that most people never face in a lifetime in a short 8 years. Samantha is now 10 years old and entering 5th grade. She is a well-adjusted pre-teen girl. We have worked hard to advocate for her and now we are working hard to help her develop her own advocacy skills so that she will succeed in situations that she will face throughout her adult life.

I teach an advocacy class to parents based on my training from Wrightslaw. Here are my top ten tips for advocating for your child:

10. Educate yourself about the legal rights of deaf/hard of hearing children.

9. Get to know your IEP team members, it's much easier to work out differences with people when you know more about them.

8. Create and build strong, lasting relationships with your school personnel—they're the ones who will be working with your child on a regular basis.

7. Make your child aware of their needs, as they get older they will become more involved in the IEP process.

6. Speak to your spouse or partner to make sure you are both on common ground before meetings.

5. Have two lists; the "Must Have" list and the "Wish" list. Be willing to forgo items from the wish list to get items from the must have list.

4. Be very clear on what you're asking from the team and the teachers.

3. Start working on your child's self advocacy skills, he/she is going to need them for the rest of his/her life, start NOW.

2. Don't rush into any decisions you are not comfortable with. Take some time to review before moving ahead.

And the # 1 tip: Take time for yourself!

Raising Skip

~ Sue Flanagan

It is almost inconceivable that no two people in the world are alike, but it is what makes life so exciting. Our journey raising a deaf son was not expected, but has been an amazing, fulfilling life experience. Every parent is challenged with making the best decisions for their child in order for them to grow, develop and ultimately reach their potential. As parents of a deaf son, we have busy lives filled with tears, fears, laughter, hopes and dreams like every parent, we just do things differently.

Skip was identified with severe sensori-neural hearing loss at 17 months old. We had long suspected that he was deaf. After many trips to doctors and professionals his diagnosis was finally confirmed. We realized then he was still the same happy child we knew and loved but we now had a critical piece of information that would change our lives. We were passionate that we would focus on raising our son, free from labels and help him to reach his dreams. We knew we would face challenging issues but we knew we were not alone. We have met amazing professionals, incredible families and life - long friends that we would not have met if not for our son.

One of the most valuable resources for us are the members of the Deaf community. They are a tremendous source of support and direction. It was important for us that Skip interact and communicate with other members of the Deaf community as he grew up regardless of his educational choices or whether he was using his hands and/or voice. This is a community that understood us.

Skip, now a first year student at Rochester institute of Technology attended a school for the deaf for Pre-K through elementary, a regional mainstreamed program for the deaf for middle school and utilizing an interpreter, he attended a private Catholic high school. American Sign Language is Skip's first language.

Skip experienced a diverse educational background in which he was involved in most all decisions--because it was critical to us that he know how to represent and advocate for himself.

Skip, now a young adult, tries to make the world more respectful of those with different abilities, and has instructed hundreds of hearing students in American Sign Language and deaf culture. He believes the world's true wealth lie in the abilities and uniqueness of each individual and he sees the best in everyone. He respects differences and promotes tolerance. Having a cousin with autism who is non-verbal, Skip has grown up with examples of unconditional love, advocacy and patience all around him. These are truly the values we believe all children are deserving of. Skip is steadfast in his personal goals and maintains an incredible sense of humor about life. Being deaf is only one of many characteristics that define him.

Skip's passion in life is playing baseball. From playing T-ball to now being a two-way player of the RIT varsity baseball team, Skip experienced many life lessons through this sport. He often commented that the baseball diamond was a level playing field where language was secondary to athletic performance and competitive spirit. Sports have historically offered many metaphors for life. Having experienced many different coaches and multitudes of teammates he has learned how to compete, stay focused, and seek excellence.

Every year during tryouts, Skip would do his best and then we would wait to hear if he successfully made the team. The anticipation was always stressful. We told him that if he did not make the team because his performance wasn't his best, he must accept it BUT if he did not make the team because of his deafness, he should never accept it. Knowing the difference would always be challenging, so he must always bring his best game. Learning to face challenges and those who don't believe in your potential are part of life. Having self confidence and living your dream should be a way of life.

For us, life is not about what you have or don't have, it is most importantly about using the gifts God has given us. We have tried to teach and model for Skip: live each day to its fullest, be the best person you can be, and share your gifts with the world every day. We know he has touched many lives, most of all ours. I think as parents, we think the sole responsibility for teaching lies with us when in fact, our children have a lot to teach us. We have learned a lot.

We believe God doesn't make mistakes and we personally feel blessed He chose us to be Skip's parents. Though the journey of raising a deaf child may have felt overwhelming at moments, we have unlimited treasured memories. It has been the best journey of our lives............ it still is!

Chapter 8
The Social Stuff

Everybody laughs the same in every language because laughter is a universal connection.

~ Yakov Smirnoff

One of my biggest concerns when my kids were growing up was their connection with their peers. When they were little, the peer stuff was easy. I'd drag them to the mall with other moms of deaf and hard of hearing kids. We attended deaf and hard of hearing events. Then off to the park to play with the neighbor kids, all who could hear a bird chirp a mile away. We attended regular play dates in the neighborhood as well. Then there was our monthly Mothers of Preschoolers program where they were able to hang out with 20 other kids while I soaked up some intelligent conversation from other frazzled moms and worked on a craft.

When it came to elementary school, I took the approach of "Bloom where you're planted" because my kids were the only deaf and hard of hearing kids in their school. I volunteered in the classroom and at the school library so I could get to know the other moms and the school staff. And here's the thing, when kids are really young, it's easy to get them all to bond. They have one thing on their mind: play.

And kids, when they're young, they're open and curious. Many of the kids picked up a few signs from the interpreter and they loved using those signs to interact with my kids. They didn't hold back on their questions. "What can you hear? What are those things in your ears?"

As they became older, the social stuff became more of a challenge in different ways. The conversations became more sophisticated. The other kids became less willing to make accommodations in group conversations. So Joe and I doubled up our efforts to connect our kids with other deaf and hard of hearing peers. We did social events, camps and sleepovers.

In the process of writing this book, my daughter reminded me to share an important point of hers. Just because two kids are deaf/hard of hearing doesn't mean they're going to connect as friends. She's got a point. This means you have to cast an even wider net to meet deaf and hard of hearing kids to see if they'll connect with your own kid/s!

Even as an adult, the social stuff is a challenge for me. I'll give you a glimpse into this by using my return to barefoot water skiing as an example.

The first time I sat in a boat with several other barefoot water skiers there was the awkward dance of getting to know each other. Keith, the instructor, usually remembered to look at me and he slowed down his speech so I could lipread him. There was a funny moment on the water when he yelled at the top of his lungs, only to realize the futility of it all; with or without hearing aids, hollering is useless.

The challenge always comes with multiple people in one place—the conversations always flow faster than the eyes can keep up. Thus, the game of social ping pong comes into play. It starts with lipreading one person, then zipping to the next one and the next one. By the time one person says something, the other one answers and a third one chimes in, the deaf/hard of hearing person is lost.

It takes time for people to get used to the communication challenges when talking with me. I've been fortunate in some situations where one person will summarize a group conversation if I'm lost.

There are times when we've had to get creative with communication. For example, Keith will face me when giving instructions to another skier so I can lipread him and learn at the same time. Once, when he had to stand behind me to teach me a new skill, he had another skier repeat everything in front of me so I could lipread what was said. Other times, he has used the iPhone to type out instructions or communicate.

I've also been in situations where I've asked someone to summarize and they say, "Oh, you didn't miss anything."

Ouch. That always hurts. Most of the time I explain how I feel and I ask them once again to summarize. They usually "get it" at that point.

People often don't have an understanding of what I miss out on. And because I can't hear it, I don't know I'm missing out on stuff around me.

At a recent barefoot tournament banquet, I brought in two interpreters to translate for two hours. A lot of folks were surprised. That was an "ah-ha" moment for many of them to realize just how "deaf" I really am. The interpreters ensure me access to most of what's going on. I don't have to fight to lipread everyone around me. I don't have to struggle to fill in the words I miss when lipreading. I don't have to wonder what they're saying at the podium.

Remember my earlier advice? Whatever it takes. Get creative and make the communication bridges happen for your kid/s.

The Schmidt Family: An Adoption Story

~Susan Schmidt

My husband and I have adopted six children. Two through domestic adoption, and four children were placed in our family through international adoption from Russia. Our adopted children's ages range from three to 22 years old.

Our son, Gregory, was 12 months old when he joined our family from Russia thirteen years ago. At 21 months old, he started raging, and lost his ability to understand what he heard (auditory processing) and his ability to speak. We suspected a possible delayed reaction to the vaccinations he received in Russia – perhaps too many in too short of a time for his small body. At 12 months old, he was the size of a seven-month old baby, but he soon caught up to normal growth. At four and half years old, he lost his hearing and became deaf. Tests showed a genetic cause. I told God, that I could deal with deafness. What I could not deal with was the raging. It took a lot of patience and guidance, but Gregory eventually ceased the raging.

Our family began the process of learning about deaf kids, deaf programs in schools, sign language, hearing aids, hearing tests, cochlear implants, and speech therapy. Our family went to sign language classes at the local colleges and at the deaf program schools. We even had private classes in our home for awhile. We are all intermediate signers.

Over the next three years, Gregory was able to learn to speak, even though he could not hear the sounds of speech with his hearing aids. At nine years old, he received a cochlear implant. After a lot of speech therapy, it was concluded that he doesn't have a good long term auditory memory. This we believe is related to his early auditory processing problem. But his speech continued to improve. Before the implant, he spoke words and afterwards, he spoke in sentences. Sign language still remains his first language.

Because of our contact with the deaf community, we received information about a deaf boy in Russia. The email was from a woman searching for a family for him. We thought we were finished adopting children, but we felt if God wanted us to do this, we would look into it. When we inquired about six-year-old Luke, we were told that other families were interested in him. Then later, the agency called to say that the other families had to back out for various reasons. We decided to pursue the adoption of this little boy. It felt so much easier to think about adopting a deaf child now because of our experience with Gregory. Looking back, I remember how hard it was finding out that Gregory was deaf and we had so much to learn. But this time around, we were confident as parents of a deaf son.

We wanted Luke to have a sibling closer in age than Gregory, who was 12 at the time, so we inquired if there was another deaf child available in the region. The agency told us about an 18-month old little girl, Annie, who was deaf in one ear and had hearing loss in the other. We were hoping for a boy who was a few years younger than Luke, but again, God had something else in mind for us. We felt led to pursue the adoption of both children.

After some paper work, we were allowed to visit both children in Russia for five days. We were concerned how Luke would interact with us, since he had no language.

Every day, we visited Luke in the morning and Annie in the afternoon. He was delighted to visit with us and began learning signs right away. He was eager to please us and loved all the attention we gave him. We visited Annie, almost two years old, in the baby orphanage. At that time, we were told that Annie had normal hearing in one ear and was deaf in the other ear. She was so afraid and so unresponsive, I was concerned about her. After a few days, a smile would peek out. By Friday, she was laughing and interacting with me. I was amazed at the transformation. She understood what the Russians said to her, but did not speak. I believe that she was experiencing "failure to thrive", having lived her whole life in the hospital and then the orphanage with no one to nurture her. The head doctor later told me that she really changed after we came to visit. I say she "came to life". We brought Luke to meet Annie and they immediately connected. Annie seemed to be comfortable with Luke. We fell in love with both kids and couldn't wait to bring them home.

The following winter, we completed all our paperwork, our court date was set, and we were able to return. It was four months since we were there, and I was worried that Annie would forget me. But she walked into my open arms and seemed happy to see me. She was still wary of men and slow to connect with my husband, which is very common in orphanages where the staff is mostly female.

Luke was excited to see us. We went to court and my husband flew back home. We had to wait 10 days before the adoption decree would be granted. I chose to stay to spend the time with the children, visiting them every day, teaching Luke sign language and getting to know him, and helping Annie become more confident before we had to fly home.

Once we were home, it really surprised me how happy they both were. Luke seemed to appreciate the freedom of having no schedule, being able to play outside when he wanted to. Annie was so happy on the plane trips home, in the car in Moscow, in the hotel. She sang little nonsense songs--babbling with a melody. She didn't care where she was as long as I was with her. Both of them just basked in all the attention they received from their new parents and siblings. I was surprised at how quickly Luke bonded to Annie. They do have an attachment with each other and play together.

Now, Luke and Annie have been home for a year. Luke is profoundly deaf, has a cochlear implant, is doing well in school in the deaf program, and he reads simple stories. He has a good imagination, enjoys being read to, and playing games. His language skills are improving every day. We were pleasantly surprised to learn Annie has normal hearing in both ears. When she hears loud sounds, though, she freezes rather than looking in the direction of the sound. It is not too surprising that she didn't respond well to their hearing tests. She doesn't do this much anymore. Both children are thriving in our home and we are so happy to have them here.

Chapter 9
Born to Stand Out

Why are you trying so hard to fit in when you were born to stand out?

~ From the movie, *What a Girl Wants*

The first time I came across the quote above I immediately looked back on my life and wished that someone had told me that when I was in elementary school. From the moment I received my first hearing aid at the age of nine, I hid it. I hated that thing.

I did my best to fit in, blend in, and fly under the radar. I created elaborate systems to make this happen. I became the Queen of Bluffing– learning how to laugh at the right moment and nod along in conversation– all without understanding a thing.

I developed elaborate strategies to get through the school day. "Hey, I was spacing out, what's the homework?" I'd ask the student next to me. In English class, the teacher had us read paragraphs from a book– I'd count the number of students ahead of me, watch each of them like hawk to see where they finished each paragraph and then when it was my turn, I knew where to start reading. If there was a discussion, I made sure to chime in with my opinion first. I couldn't follow the conversation and as long as I was first, it meant that I wouldn't say something that was already said.

When my own kids started sporting hearing aids, we picked some "stand out" colors so that there was no mistaking the ornaments perched in their ears. Lauren and I picked out matching earmolds one year– pink glitter for her and blue glitter for me. And to my surprise, even after all my efforts of getting my kids comfortable with being deaf and hard of hearing, they still went through their own journey of wanting to fit in, blend in and fly under the radar. The wild colors were replaced with plain, clear earmolds. Hair grew over their ears. The boys went through a stage of long hair. For all three kids, this transition happened during the middle school years. I had to learn to back off as a mom and let them experience their journey their own way. Soon enough, they became comfortable again in standing out, but not with their hearing aids-- it was with their signing. The oldest two joined a deaf drama group, the same one that launched Marlee Matlin's acting career.

I think back to my elementary and teen years– I spent way too much time trying to be a poor imitation of a person who could hear instead of the best "me" I could be.

When I was a teen, I took a fall while barefoot water skiing and in an instant, I went from hard of hearing to deaf. I could no longer hear any sounds without my hearing aid. I was forced to wear the contraption 24/7.

I was miserable at first. This sudden turn in life brought many nights of tears and a lot of struggle.

This is one of the reasons becoming deaf turned out to be a blessing for me; I learned how to be the best possible me. I finally became comfortable at showing the world the vibrant, beautiful *deaf* part of me.

And you know what I wish I had more of while I was growing up? Deaf and hard of hearing role models. It's one thing to see them on TV or read about them in a book, but a whole other ballgame to have an adult in your life who can mentor, guide and shape you while growing up.

I will never forget the mom who came to a Parent Connection meeting that I hosted at a nearby school. The mom stood up and related a conversation that she had with her young son before bed one night. Her son said, "Mom, when I grow up, I want to be a fireman!" The mom's voice started to break. She simply agreed with him, "Deep down, I knew he could never be a fireman with his hearing loss," she said. "It made me sad for him."

What I shared next hit her like a ton of bricks.

"Here's the thing... I know a fireman who works at a local fire department and he is deaf," I told her. "I know a volunteer fireman out east who is also deaf."

The mom's face lit up. I will never forget the amazement on her face. Her son's world had just opened up.

That's why role models are so important. Of course, it's easy to find the ones in the news who are doing amazing things. Ashley Fiolek is all over the sports arena as the top female motorcross rider. Marlee Matlin is a well-known Hollywood star. Matt Hamill is a pro boxer featured on ESPN many times. Vin Cerf is the father of the Internet and now the Vice President of Google. Yes, they're deaf or hard of hearing. And... there are so many deaf and hard of hearing folks out there who are quietly doing their jobs every day.

Now let me ask you, what do these four folks have in common?

Charles Henri Nicolle
Sir Charles Scott Sherrington
Sir John Warcup Cornforth
Dr. Andrew Manning

Most likely, you probably have never seen their names before. Their names aren't familiar to most of us. All four of them are scientists who won the Nobel Peace Prize. All four are deaf/hard of hearing.

Here are some that I'd like to share:

Jessica Haung is a pharmacist. She interned at Walgreens and her first job was with Kaiser Permanente in California, specializing in cancer care. She's currently consulting in her field.

Dr. Carolyn Stern is a doctor. When a dean in college tried to discourage her from being a doctor, Carolyn chose not to listen. Dr. Stern started out catching babies at Lutheran General hospital in Illinois and today, she has a family practice in Rochester, New York. She has been featured in People magazine.

Greg Gunderson is a race car driver. When he was six, (yes, six-years-old!!) he signed himself up for a snowmobile race and won against older, experienced kids. He began racing cars in high school. He has done over 750 sprint car races and has a room full of trophies.

Dr. Tom McDavitt had a love for animals since he was a kid. He wanted to be a veterinarian. Several tried to discourage him. He persisted in his dream and today, he is the owner of The Animal Clinic in Alsip, Illinois.

Karen Meyer is a news reporter at ABC News in Chicago. She reports on disability issues and is on the news two times a week. She's been doing this for 21 years. She also teaches at DePaul University and has her own consulting firm.

Brenda Stoltz is the CEO of Ariad Partners, a consulting firm that provides business strategies for 5 million to 200 million dollar companies. She teaches Marketing, Social Media and Business classes at Northern Virginia Community College.

Kenny Killian is a personal trainer who works in a gym teaching folks how to sculpt their bodies with weights and proper food.

Tate Tullier grabbed his mother's camera as a kid and he hasn't let go of a camera since then. Today, he flies all over doing photo shoots and runs his own photography business. www.tatetullier.com

Cynthia Murray started her own business from home, 4Legz, an organic dog treat business. Her business is booming so much that she quit her job and now does this full-time.

Sean Forbes grew up in a house filled with music. His parents gave him a drum set when he was five, and a dream was born right then and there: he wanted to make a career out of music. Sean just released his first album, *Perfect Imperfection*.

Melody and Russ Stein own Mozzeria, an Italian pizzeria restaurant in San Francisco, California. Most of their staff are also deaf and hard of hearing. Some customers are oblivious to this fact, as one reviewer thought they were just gesturing Italians.

Dr. Steven Rattner and Dr. Bo Buyn: Both dentists operate their practice together at two offices in Maryland.

Leslie Carothers owns Kaleidoscope Partnership, a social media agency specializing in the furniture business. She partners with Kathy Ireland on projects.

Stephen Hopson was the first deaf person to become an instrument-rated pilot. He is a speaker and the author of "Obstacle Illusions."

Chris Littlewood is a Project Coordinator at the St. Petersburg College's Center for Public Safety Innovation and the National Terrorism Preparedness Institute. He designs and delivers training for our nation's emergency and first responders, the military, and the public.

Ken Arcia is the social media manager for AT & T. He has Neurofibromatosis, Type II and became deaf at age 21. He's the recipient of the I. King Jordan Distinguished Service award and serves on the board of DeafHope.

Deborah Mayer is the owner of Crossroads Solution Coaching. She's a professional certified coach with training in leadership coaching at Georgetown University and Adler Professional School of Coaching-Arizona and is recognized by the International Coach Federation (ICF).

Joel Barish is an entrepreneur who has always created opportunities in his life. He's the host of "No Barriers," a documentary-style show where he travels the world and showcases deaf folks from all walks of life. He and his brother, Jed, run the Deaf Nation trade shows in major cities.

Mark Sorokin is a lawyer. He holds degrees from Johns Hopkins University and University of Arizona. He runs a private practice, Sorokin Law Offices, focusing on estate planning.

Susan Lacke is a no-meat triathlete and a columnist for The Competitor and Triathlete magazine. She holds a Masters and PhD in Health and Wellness.

And to quote Susan:

"Case in point: I'm deaf. I've spent most of my life being told I can't do a lot of things because of my disability. I guarantee you, it hasn't stopped me from doing a single thing...except (maybe) hurt my chances of ever becoming the next "American Idol." But I'll be damned if I don't sing off-key in my car anyway."

Yes, all of the above folks are deaf or hard of hearing. Each of them had a passion, a desire, a path... and went out and pursued it. It didn't matter that they didn't have the complete sense of hearing. What mattered is that they believed in themselves, they beat the odds, and they overcame the naysayers.

Now let me tell you about Mark Levin. This guy had a burning desire to play music. He picked up a guitar when he was eight and his passion for music was born. Never mind that he couldn't hear all the notes, he loved to create new songs. When Mark sat down with his vocational rehabilitation counselor to plan for college, he was clear on his goals: he wanted a music degree and a career in the field. His counselor disagreed. "There's a certain path for deaf kids from high school to college," said Mark's mom, Shirley. "Mark wasn't a cookie cutter kid. I don't feel his career options were open for him. It's either 'this way' or 'that way'—there was no real career coaching either."

Mark held fast to his dreams and declined the full vocational rehabilitation ride at a college for deaf students. Instead, he took two, and sometimes three, different jobs to put himself through Columbia College. He graduated with a degree in business music production and another degree in education. Today, he writes music and tours full-time with deaf musician Sean Forbes.

"In a typical situation, there's an attitude of 'you're deaf, how will you do that?'" said Shirley. "I hate to hear that and Mark does too. Mark can't hear like a normal person, but there's nothing wrong with him. Nothing."

Early this summer, one of David's friends, Ronnie Cuartero stopped at our house on his Bike Across America trip. I was totally amazed by this young man. He first planned to bike from Rochester, New York to San Francisco, California along with several other deaf friends. One by one, they each dropped out of the plan. Ronnie remained dedicated to the goal and decided to bike the trip by himself.

Solo.

2,650 miles.

Solo.

By the time Ronnie arrived at our house, he had biked 600 miles. He regaled us with stories of the people he met along the way, the sites and the challenges he encountered along the way. Never mind the fact that he can't use his voice to speak, Ronnie always found a way to communicate with everyone he met on the journey.

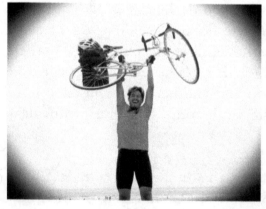

When he left our house, Ronnie was facing a possible detour in Colorado due to the forest fires, but he was determined to accomplish his dream. He didn't have any sponsors, nor was he riding for a cause; he was doing it to challenge himself. To see what he was made of.

"I want to be able to look back and say, 'I did it!'" he said.

It took him 52 days to reach Ocean Beach, California but he did it.

And in case you accuse me of being a Pollyanna and sugar-coating this whole "Deaf and hard of hearing people can do anything stuff," I will say this:

Yeah, the road is going to be tough, no matter what. Your kid is going to face discrimination. There will be people out there who put up barriers. Heck, there will be barriers, no matter what. But it comes down to this: maybe your kid has to blaze the way. Maybe *your* kid will be the first to do something no one else has done.

Along the journey, we've faced challenges as a family.

As a kid, David loved baseball. He started playing T-ball when he was four and his first coach happened to be the father of a deaf daughter. He coaxed David to develop his skills and gave him a great start in the sport. Over the years, David had a variety of coaches and his skills continued to grow.

One year, we had a coach who was very competitive. At first, everything looked good. He played David in a variety of positions and made every effort to communicate with him. Little by little, things began to change. David began to sit on the bench more and more when his teammates were out in the field. Yet, David kept his turn at bat and he was delivering results. As the games stretched on and the bench warming became more frequent, I started to fume. My husband noticed the same thing, but he was reluctant to read too much into it. A few more games later, we couldn't deny what was happening and it was starting to affect David's self esteem on the team. He couldn't figure out why the coach wasn't playing him on the field.

My gut instinct was telling me the coach was letting the "deaf stuff" get in the way. We studied the statistic sheets and there it was in black and white—my kid was sitting out far more than any other kid on the team. Yet he was batting one of the highest in the league.

I stopped at the coach's house after a game and expressed my concerns about David sitting out so much. He hemmed and hawed and tried to sidestep the whole issue, but he finally admitted the truth: he wasn't playing David because he couldn't hear his instructions when he was out on the field. Needless to say, that coach never worked with David after that season and we made sure he could not draft David on any of his future teams. David went on to a traveling team with great coaches after that.

In Lauren's case, we faced a challenge in first grade. On her early tests, she scored in the gifted range (97th to 99th percentile) except on the auditory parts of the test. Her teacher recommended her for the gifted program, but the gifted program teacher denied her access. I explained the impact of her hearing loss and the auditory portion of the test, but she was not convinced. During a meeting to discuss the situation, the teacher from the gifted program said to me, "I don't see enough to indicate placement in the gifted program." Yet, Lauren scored just as high (with the exception of the auditory portion) as her best friend, who was in the program.

We decided not to pursue the issue any further. Life hummed along and Lauren continued to do very well in school. By third grade, the teachers were recommending placement in the gifted program for fourth grade. At first, things went well. Lauren enjoyed the challenge. As the school year went on, she became miserable. She felt the teacher was condescending and the friction began to build up. I expressed my concern to the team--but I didn't listen to that little voice inside of me which nagged at me. Something was wrong. In fifth grade, things became worse. Lauren didn't want to go to school and she was having frequent emotional swings. I chalked it up to pre-teen hormones, even though she expressed her displeasure with the gifted teacher.

Things finally came to a head one morning and Lauren broke down crying. I decided right then and there—we had enough. It was time to make some changes even though we had just two months of school left. I pulled her out of the gifted program and literally overnight, she was a changed kid. It had nothing to do with the work in the program, but everything to do with the teacher. In middle school, she tested back into the gifted program and she loved it there. I learned not to ignore that gut feeling. When you feel something is wrong, listen within.

Now on to another challenge; this one involved me and Steven. The two of us drove through a local drive-thru and we wanted to order two milkshakes. I pulled right up to the window to give my order. The employee insisted I had to drive around again and use the speaker to place the order. I explained that I was deaf and couldn't hear. He continued to insist it was company policy and he wanted us to go around again. We argued at the window—I couldn't believe how the situation was unfolding. I explained about the Americans with Disabilities Act and how going up to the window was an accommodation under the law. As it ended up, we never did get our milkshakes. The guy refused to serve us and threatened to call the cops for "holding up the drive-thru line."

And all we wanted was two milkshakes. Heck, we were willing to give them money too!

"Did you do something wrong?" Steven asked me as we pulled away. "Why is he calling the police?" I reassured him we did nothing wrong. The incident ended up on blogs everywhere as well as newspapers and on TV. Fortunately, the restaurant made some policy changes and instituted training for their employees.

Yup, there will always be those bumps in the road along the journey!

Getting Involved with Deaf and Hard of Hearing Adults.

I can't stress this enough; deaf and hard of hearing kids benefit greatly when they have deaf and hard of hearing adults in their lives. Even if you live in a rural area with no other deaf/hard of hearing kids/adults around for miles-- the Internet is an amazing place. Head out to the library if you don't have access at home. YouTube is filled with thousands of inspirational videos produced by deaf and hard of hearing folks. Google is your best friend. In fact, you can go to Google.com and set up a Google Alert for the words, "deaf" and "hard of hearing" and Google will email links with those topics.

Take the time to seek out deaf and hard of hearing adults and older teens. Ask them questions:

- What is/was it like growing up deaf/hard of hearing?

- What do/did you like best about school? What is/was challenging?

- What accommodations do/did you find helpful?

- What is a typical day like for you?

- What's the best part about being deaf/hard of hearing?

"Be yourself. There is something that you can do better than any other. Listen to the inward voice and bravely obey that."

~ Unknown

The following is from Mark "Drolz" Drolsbaugh, a deaf father of a deaf son. Mark is the author of three books: Deaf Again, Anything But Silent, and On the Fence. He works as a school counselor at the Pennsylvania School for the Deaf. I had the pleasure of meeting Mark and his wife for dinner one night and the guy had me in stitches with his sense of humor. But here, he shares the serious stuff:

One Size Does Not Fit All

~ Mark Drolsbaugh

There are two suggestions I have for parents of deaf/hard of hearing kids. First, keep in mind that there doesn't have to be an either/or. If anyone tells you that there's a particular communication style or technological device that must be used at the exclusion of other options, RUN. There's a continuum of communication styles. Every unique child has his or own place somewhere along this continuum. Some kids prefer one thing more than anything else, and other kids may prefer a combination. Your child will lead you to whatever works best. You'll see which approaches come naturally and which ones don't fit (sorry, one size doesn't fit all).

Second, and most important, are peers. Find other deaf/hard of hearing kids and allow opportunities for your kids to socialize with them as much as possible. One of the most maddening myths regarding deaf children is that if you allow them to interact with other deaf people, you'll "lose them to the deaf community." Nothing could be further from the truth. I have two hearing children (in addition to one deaf son) and I send them to hearing schools. Guess what? They keep coming back. I haven't lost them to the hearing culture or whatever. Likewise, the same for deaf children. If you keep your mind open and allow deaf/hard of hearing children to connect with others who are in the same boat, you'll open new doors for them. Deaf/hard of hearing role models may help immensely in getting your child to internalize a "can do" attitude. Also, a lot of deaf/hard of hearing children are stressed from the effort it takes to "fit in" the mainstream; the opportunity to be with deaf/hard of hearing peers gives them a healthy outlet, a sense of belonging that validates they're just fine exactly the way they are.

Chapter 10
Something More

Don't go through life, grow through life.

~ Eric Butterworth

In the complexities of raising kids, sometimes it's really tough to figure out what is a personality thing, what's a behavior issue and what's related to being deaf/hard of hearing. There's an excellent article about this written by Leeanne Seaver on the Hands & Voices website titled "Is This a Deaf Thing?"

(http://www.handsandvoices.org/articles/perfect/V13_3-deafthing.htm)

In the case of families who are juggling multiple disabilities or other issues, sometimes the deaf/hard of hearing stuff gets lost in the shuffle. Mindi Allen's daughter was diagnosed with cancer on the fourth day of her life and started chemotherapy the very next day. When she didn't pass the newborn hearing screening, they planned to follow up with another test a month later. Two more tests showed the same results. "We were in survival mode," Mindi recalled. "We were worried about the cancer. The hearing loss was the least of our worries. I was sad and in shock. All this time, I had been playing music and singing to her."

For two years, the cancer played out like a roller coaster for the family and finally stabilized. Mindi was fortunate to connect with another parent from the Guide By Your Side program in her state. The parent guide, Cari Piper, also had a child with an NICU experience so she gave Mindi a lot of support with her shared experience.

"In the beginning, I cried—I was a wreck," said Mindi. "We were dealing with so much at once. Cari shared her story with me. She was very open, very candid and we had an immediate connection and rapport. She helped me to see that everything would eventually be okay."

I worked with a family with a child with CHARGE syndrome and after a particularly trying week filled with countless therapy visits and doctor appointments, the mom confessed that she was just way too stressed and tired to focus on language and communication. She was feeling guilty and the guilt stressed her out even more. She felt like she had nothing left to give her child at that point. And to make matters worse, she also felt as if her child was racing against an hourglass of time and the sand was pouring down. The "window of opportunity" for her child to optimize the language development was closing in on her.

The antidote? A little fun.

If Mom and Dad are stressed, frazzled and worn out, chances are, the kid is too. More often than not, therapy and doctor appointments are "work" for the kid. That's when it's time to pull back a bit. Get a sitter and take an evening out. If you don't let go and take care of *you*, then you won't be in top condition to take care of anything or anyone else. Do something different and fun as a family. Find the joy.

Raising Paula

~ Juliet Martinez

Paula was a sensitive baby who cried a lot, then around five months of age she started shrieking all the time. If she was happy, she shrieked. If she was cold, she shrieked. If she was frustrated, she shrieked. It went on all day, and she didn't like to take naps or go to sleep, so I listened to this shrieking from early in the morning until nine or ten at night.

My doctor at the time recommended I wear Paula in the sling more, which I was already doing a lot, and give her time. I asked for a hearing screening since Paula had missed her newborn screening, but first one doctor and later others insisted she was fine, she just needed time.

I became so frazzled from spending all my time with this tiny shrieking infant that I began to fantasize about being killed in a car accident. I knew I needed help, but when I went to a therapist to talk about what I was feeling, she accused me of blaming Paula for my problems. I suppose it was actually the fault of doctors and that therapist, none of whom offered anything to help my situation. But now I know anyone who has a baby like Paula struggles mightily to feel sane and just survive that first year.

Once Paula's hearing loss was diagnosed at 19 months, I became focused on helping her learn to sign, and eventually to learn English. My life took on an additional level of intensity as I became her gateway to all the world's information. And as I powered through every day learning new signs with Paula, fingerspelling everything I couldn't sign, trying to bring the world in through her eyes, I was still really struggling with my own emotional state. Around the time Paula turned two she began to wake up in the middle of the night and stay awake for hours at a time. This disrupted my sleep dramatically, further destabilizing my emotions. When Paula was almost two and a half, I got a prescription for antidepressants.

After that my depression surged up around my head at times of change, especially when I had big decisions to make about Paula's schooling. I felt overwhelmed by my responsibility to educate my child who seemed to need so much. In contrast, the decision to homeschool was easier for me than most of the previous educational transitions. It really felt right.

We started homeschooling after Paula's first grade year. During kindergarten she had repeatedly expressed her wish to be in a school where there were other deaf and hard of hearing kids. She didn't like being the only one with hearing aids, she got tired of people asking her what was in her ears, and she wanted some friends who knew how to sign. I felt it would be good for her to have those things, so we moved her to a school with a deaf program.

In the first place, Paula didn't get along with the other deaf kids. She was much more able to express herself whether in sign language or English, and she couldn't talk with them about any of her interests in Harry Potter, fairies, mermaids and all things imaginary. Her social skills were not up to par with either hearing or deaf peers, and she had trouble making friends. She was advanced in reading relative to her hearing peers and as a result spent a good deal of time bored in her mainstream class. Add to that her poor impulse control and focus, and she was in trouble a lot. Her teacher did not try to give Paula extra activities to ameliorate her boredom, but mainly focused on Paula's bad behavior. It was a difficult year. At home Paula had meltdowns three or four afternoons a week after school, and Sunday afternoons were the worst. She never failed to have such an extreme tantrum on Sundays that I put them on the calendar in advance, reminding myself to feed her a good lunch and give her a hot bath to try to calm her. At times she even became aggressive toward me and her little brother, who at that time was under a year old.

When the school year ended, I saw her change. She began to relax and connect more with me, her brother and her dad. I just knew I couldn't send her back to the school where she had gone for first grade, and it was too late in the year for me to move her. So I kept her home. The decision was easily made, though the actual homeschooling was a challenge. In the end we haven't done much academic work, just reading a lot and following Paula's curiosity. The real work has been on those non-academic and non-cognitive skills where she was lagging far behind, and family therapy played a major role.

The therapist focused on giving us tools to use as a family. It was short-term therapy, so every session involved discussing a problem, talking about some concrete approaches to that problem, and then making sure we agreed on one and understood it well enough to try it out in real life, so to speak.

The therapist first got us all to practice "cooling off" when emotions flared. So Paula's meltdowns were handled by asking her to cool off, but when Joel and I got frustrated with her for ignoring us or mouthing off, we had to go cool off, too. After that, the therapist worked with us on building up routines that Paula would have to do throughout the day to make transitions easier. This exercise helped us enormously, and gave me the skills to institute a chore regimen for Paula that has been a source of tremendous growth for her in terms of focus, consistency and taking responsibility for our home.

We only had four or five therapy sessions, but they made a huge difference in how our family works together. And I saw that as a result of Joel and I learning some new skills, Paula really matured. She doesn't have big meltdowns anymore, transitions are much easier. I can think of a few things we could get more help with, but nothing is urgent now like it was a year ago.

Now Paula is asking to go to school next year, and I think with a year of advance notice we will be able to find a good school for her. Her character is improving and I see her growing into her imaginative nature in a healthy, positive way. I think she'll be ready for school next year.

I still don't really know which of the things we have dealt with as a family since Paula's birth were caused by her hearing loss. I have talked to parents of deaf and hoh kids who talked about their kids being easy babies, having an even temperament and none of the challenges Paula has faced. On the other hand professionals have told me Paul's behavior issues are "normal for a gifted deaf child."

So I'm stumped.

When Paula and I went to the Pre-School Institute at a state school for deaf and hard of hearing kids, nobody talked about behavioral issues that could arise as a result of communication difficulties or that might just happen alongside the child's deafness. I felt for a long time like I was the only one, but eventually I found another mom, Julie Vassilatos. She and I provided a lot of support and commiseration for each other as our daughters stormed through our lives like class five hurricanes.

Things have gotten a lot better for Paula. For us, the combination of family therapy and homeschooling have made a difference.

When Paula was little I was fixated on teaching her as much language as I could, learning signs for everything imaginable, and fingerspelling anything I didn't know how to sign. I provided non-stop narration of where we were, what we were doing, what everything was called, and as much about the world as I could get into her sightline. But I neglected to focus enough on her social and emotional skills, or put another way, her character development. Sending her to preschool before age three seemed like the best thing to do at the time, but we sure missed out on developing her non-cognitive and non-academic areas; our family paid for that later.

It's a catch-22, though: how can a child develop emotionally without the ability to express herself? How can she be lovingly taught how to interact with others if she lacks the basic language skills to ask for something or find out why she's been put in time-out?

Maybe it doesn't have to be either language or character. Maybe if I had it to do all over again I would keep her at home longer, do the organized activities on a part-time basis, and work on social skills more at that early age.

But of course if I had it to do over again I would be a different person. Back when Paula was a toddler I was so blown away by her sheer intensity, her non-stop tantrums, her neediness, her complete resistance to sleep, and my own profound bereavement at the loss of the motherhood I had envisioned. I was depressed, overwhelmed and barely staying afloat. I don't blame myself for doing what I did - not only did I do my best, but Paula is a terrific kid, not just extremely bright but also creative, loving and loyal. And through homeschooling I have been able to go back in time, in a sense, and really work with her on those interpersonal and character skills that we skipped blindly over in our pursuit of her acquisition of language.

So maybe that's my advice, not to neglect the child's character development in favor of vocabulary, grammar and syntax. A lot of parents probably don't need that advice, but I definitely could have used it back then.

Chapter 11
Where Do We Go From Here

Continuity gives us roots; change gives us branches, letting us stretch and grow and reach new heights.

~ Pauline R. Kezer

In the twenty years of raising my kids, I've seen a lot of changes over the years. Back when my journey began with David, there was no Internet in my home. There was no way to Google the answers to everything. No way to instantly connect with another parent, professional or deaf/hard of hearing adult across the globe.

Yeah, we had it rough back then. Kind of like the days when our own parents had to trudge 2.5 miles to school in the snow.

Technology keeps changing at a rapid pace and it seems like every day brings something new to the table. I marvel at all the different ways my kids can connect with their peers—hearing, deaf or hard of hearing—it doesn't matter. My kids can sit at the kitchen table and chat with six other kids through ooVoo. Texting is the norm. Facebook and Twitter are their social arenas. The playing field for communication is far more level than it was when I was growing up. Back then, I had to depend on my friends to make phone calls to my boyfriend in high school. Today, I can use an interpreter on a videophone to translate conversations over the phone. Thanks to technology, I've interviewed people from all over the world for my articles and books.

In my family, there are five generations of relatives who are deaf and hard of hearing. Every now and then, a discussion would come up among us—what if there was a non-surgical solution to restoring hearing?   I recently came across an article sent to me via my blog, about the first stem cell clinical trials being done in Houston, Texas.   I also came across an article opposing the research.

I got in touch with the research team to find out more about using stem cells to restore hearing.   The idea of using stem cells to restore hearing first came about from a casual conversation between Linda Baumgartner and her husband, neurosurgeon Dr. James Baumgartner. "Jim did a few other studies with stem cells for other issues and I asked him, 'Is this something we can do for babies with hearing loss?" said Linda.   Jim was working on a trial using bone marrow for patients with traumatic brain injuries and he was intrigued with Linda's idea so he did some research and talked to several researchers.

Dr. Baumgartner came across research done in Italy that showed successful results using mice.   "The study used infant mice and exposed them to noise, antibiotics, or both-- to create hearing loss," he said.   "All of the mice were injected with human stem cells through the abdomen.   The damaged hair cells grew again—the nerves reconnected. The cells from the human cord blood triggered the mice's own hair cells to grow again."

The FDA approved a license for the first human trials on ten patients, ages six months to eighteen months. Children's Memorial Hermann Hospital in Houston, Texas and Cord Blood Registry(r) (CBR) identified two babies to receive the treatment. The first baby, whose hearing loss resulted from CMV exposure, received the first stem cell infusion on January 23, 2012.

I asked Dr. Baumgartner about the side effects from stem cell treatments and he assured me that the procedure had a strong safety record. "Safety is our goal. People are often scared of stem cell research—they freak out," he explained. "Autologous blood, giving people back their own blood products, is safe."

Once the trial shows results with at least five infants, the team can request FDA approval for the second phase which will allow an increase dosage of stem cells. The third phase would include double-blind random trials. "I feel my hypothesis is strong and I'm hopeful we will get good results," said Dr. Baumgartner.

In a discussion with a friend, she revealed that she was scared about the potential success of the stem cell trials. "It scares me to think that we would lose the beauty of deaf and hard of hearing people in the world. The world would be so bland without that diversity," she said. "Think of how the world would be without the contributions of Beethoven... or Edison... or Vint Cerf—the father of the internet. They are all deaf and hard of hearing and they contributed something valuable to the world."

My own feelings were very mixed on this. I spent the last twenty six years getting really comfortable with myself after going from hard of hearing to deaf. In sharp contrast to the teen who hid every sign of hearing loss, the teen who became deaf at nineteen learned to embrace a whole new world that included American Sign Language. My world truly opened up after becoming deaf and I saw the change as a blessing. I learned to embrace the gift I was given.

I asked Dr. Baumgartner about research on families like mine—five generations due to a mitochondrial gene. My daughter will pass this gene on to her children. He explained that bone marrow trials may be promising. "Your own bone marrow won't work. If you use a different person's blood, one without the genetic cause, another person's bone marrow would allow the organ of corti to repair itself," he said.

Talking to Dr. Baumgartner on the phone using an interpreter and learning about the possibility of growing new hair cells—like I said, this brought on mixed feelings. On one hand, there was the excitement at the possibility of progress, of being able to restore hearing. I thought of my siblings—I know each and every one of them would jump at the chance of being able to hear again.

I asked my daughter how she felt. "I want deaf kids," she said. "It makes me kind of sad to think of the world without deaf and hard of hearing people in it."

Yes, deep inside of me, there was a bit of sadness. I believe the world is a more vibrant, colorful place with the tapestry of deaf and hard of hearing people who have crossed my path over the years. I cannot imagine a world without them.

Chapter 12
Letting Go

There are two lasting bequests we can give our children. One is roots. The other is wings.

~ Hodding Carter, Jr.

"I'm done," said a weary parent. "I'm just so done. I can't believe I've finally attended my last IEP meeting."

Betsy Abou Ezzi *thought* she was done. But in reality, the battle had shifted to her son, Tony. He chose a college which was unfamiliar with providing access for deaf and hard of hearing students. He was facing a fight with the disability office in trying to obtain Real-time Captioning (CART) services for his classes.

But let me back up the story a bit. I met Betsy when her son was a junior in high school. Tony was struggling in his classes and his report card reflected mostly C's, despite his motivation to succeed and do well in school. In many of his classes, Tony was struggling to understand everything being said. Tony's self esteem began to suffer as teachers told him he was taking classes which were simply too difficult for him. His two sisters were in honors classes and getting A's. He was completely stressed out trying to keep up in his classes and his anxiety began to grow.

Computer Science was a class Tony loved, but an evaluation done by the itinerant teacher showed Tony constantly looking over at a student's computer and talking-- instead of paying attention to the teacher.

During one meeting, a guidance counselor offered a helpful suggestion: perhaps Tony could sit in a swivel chair and spin around to look at each student speaking?

"I spoke up and said that was ridiculous!" Betsy recalled.

Another professional connected me to the Abou Ezzi family and I sat down with Betsy and Tony to go over the options for his IEP. Notetakers and teacher notes, copies of Powerpoint presentations, captioning on the classroom videos and preferential seating were some of the items on his IEP.

Real-time Captioning (CART) was one of the solutions I brought up for communication access. Tony was hesitant at first. He was at the point in his life where he wanted to minimize any attention to himself in the classroom. After a bit more discussion, Tony agreed to give CART a try. The next hurdle was to get the school district to agree to the services. I attended the IEP meeting as an advocate for the family.

The meeting was an emotional one. At first, it seemed as if the IEP team was not convinced Tony needed the accommodations we requested. They produced report after report showing Tony was doing well "for a person with a hearing loss."

At this point, Betsy began crying. All the years of watching her son struggle and come home anxious were just too much. She had enough.

We discussed CART in more detail, and the team agreed to give it a try for two weeks. It took several more weeks and a little more pushing to arrange for the service.

When Tony arrived home after the first day of CART in the classroom, he expressed amazement. For the first time in his life, he realized how much information he was missing in the classroom. It all came to life on the computer screen as the captioner unfolded the words before him. He graduated from high school with all As and Bs.

Today, Tony is wrapping up his last year of law school and he's a big advocate for CART access. And yes, he was able to get the colleges to provide CART for all of his classes. He shared his thoughts about his journey:

I was born with a moderate-to-severe hearing loss which left me struggling in school to receive the same information as everyone else. When I first started to realize what my hearing loss meant, I rejected it. I wore my bulky behind-the-ear hearing aids until I was eleven—when I started to feel different from everyone else. "I want to be the same as everyone else," I told my parents. "I want to be NORMAL."

My parents would tell me, "Each and every person has something that is difficult to face, whether it is visible or not. It is what makes you unique. It is what makes you human."

I had a rough time through 8th and 9th grade, dealing with the transition from middle to high school. By the end of my freshman year, my grades were dropping far below normal. That was when I realized how much my hearing loss was affecting my education. I would respond to questions such as, "What time is it," with "Oh, sure, I know what you mean," or "Yes, I think so." I created those numerous "safe" answers but I wasn't fooling anyone.

I was blessed with luck when my Dad announced we were moving, because it gave me the chance I needed to restart my life and make better decisions about wearing hearing aids and learning to accept my disability. I could not erase the past, but I could change the future, so I decided to put a stop to my fear of my own disability and my choice forever changed what my life could and will be. By the age of 14, I started accepting my disability, but at times, I still struggle and must face difficult situations. These difficult situations do anything but stop me; they give me more self-determination, and boost my self-esteem and my goal to succeed in life.

With the help of my parents and so many others, I have developed some important strategies to deal with my hearing loss. One of these strategies is for me to become an advocate for myself, which means that it is my responsibility to seek whatever help I need from my teachers. I also discovered that I must take charge of school meetings when there are items concerning my disability that only I know, and in order to get the same education, I have to educate others about what services I need to be provided with, so that I will be on an equal playing field with receiving the same information as other students.

Much of my success in school I owe to my parents who have always fought by my side no matter what the challenge. I believe that is is the parents responsibility to research and find out what their child's disability means and how it will affect their performance/education and what services he/she will need. And the most important thing is to provide love, support and encouragement.

And finally, the road to success and knowledge is not an easy one-- no one ever said it would be--but through the challenges that you face in life, you will learn everything that there is to know about yourself... and more.

The Last IEP Meeting

My oldest child is now off to college. The last IEP meeting was bittersweet. Like Betsy, I was finally done. At the same time, I couldn't believe it was over. As a parent, you get into this mode, this rhythm year after year with your kid, and then wham-- your role is done.

There were many experiences along the way which were challenging and it wasn't always easy. I often reminded myself that it would have been the same in any environment—just different challenges– it's the nature of the journey and of life.

There were times when we questioned our decisions and explored options and considered changes. At other times we celebrated with confidence.

One of the most difficult IEP meetings we ever had was David's transition to high school. A staff member at the middle school felt strongly that we should keep him in the home district. My husband and I disagreed– we wanted David at another high school where he would have deaf and hard of hearing peers as well as a mainstreamed education. We couldn't come to an agreement at that meeting. I broke down crying at that meeting—and I've had a few of those "crying meetings" over the years with the three kids for different reasons. Fortunately, we worked out an agreement with the team and it paved the way for a smooth transition for Lauren and Steven as well.

At David's last IEP meeting, I sat and thought about all of this as I watched him talk about his experience at the "Explore Your Future" camp to the VR counselor and the district representative. I sat in awe as I watched him share his views of what he wanted for his future– this little boy of mine had turned into a young man– when did that happen?

I thought back to preschool, and how he cried during the Christmas show that the teachers put on. The teachers tried to encourage him to say his lines, but all he did was sit in his chair and cry while the other kids took turns saying and signing their lines. I look back at that time and laugh, because today I have a son who can get up on stage and put on a show now for any audience.

Go figure.

For a long time, I was the parent teaching the child–guiding David through life and sharing what I wanted him to know. Lately, I've aware the roles have shifted-- I'm learning things from my son. When we head to the gym together, he teaches me things about muscle development and he becomes my coach as he runs me through drills. "Come on Mom, you have to do one more set" he says. This all sounds a lot like the stuff I tell him at home: "Come on, clean the bathroom and sweep the living room—then you can go back to your computer game." Just yesterday, he made a stir-fry dinner while I was glued to the computer and I was surprised at how delicious it was. There he was, sharing his newly-made recipe with me and teaching *me* how to make a better stir-fry.

When I mentor families who are just starting out on the journey of raising deaf and hard of hearing kids, I'm reminded of how the beginning of the journey seems so overwhelming, so impossible, so challenging. The parents are exhausted. They just want to get through the day.

I remind them to take time to celebrate the good stuff.

"Hang on to every bit of time that you have with your child," I tell them.

Because before you know it, in the blink of an eye, all of a sudden, the last IEP meeting arrives and you will wonder how it went by so fast.

At David's high school graduation, I thought about all the people we met during his lifetime—the parents, the professionals, the deaf and hard of hearing adults—each one of them left a nugget of themselves and carved out a path for us along the way. I have two more still on the path. There will come a point where they will each take flight on their own and the parenting journey will change once again.

From Birth to Graduation, Just Like That

~ Karen Putz

In a few days, my oldest son will be marching across the stage and ending the final chapter on his high school years. I'm pretty sure I'll be sitting in an auditorium seat, crying.

There was another time not too long ago when I was crying. It was a day when I was overwhelmed and overtaken by three little kids. David was six at the time and he was on hurricane cycle, bouncing from one room to the next, creating havoc everywhere he went. He scrambled from one toy to the next, pausing long enough to whack his four-year-old sister upside the head when she wouldn't relinquish a toy that he wanted. Steven, the two-year-old, was having a meltdown on the floor–the consequence of being overtired and refusing to take a nap. The house was in shambles, with laundry scattered every which way on the floor. The missing laundry basket had turned into a step stool as wayward hands tried to reach a box of crayons on the kitchen counter. The lunch dishes sat on the table with tidbits of food glued to them. The yet-unfilled school registration forms were hidden somewhere in the piles of papers on the desk.

I sat down and cried. I counted the minutes until the hubby came home to provide some much-needed relief from a day that seemed to go on forever.

My mother-in-law tried to warn me that the day would come when I would look back on this and miss those days. "Life goes by faster and faster as the kids get older," she told me.

"Hang on to these days, because before you know it, they'll be over with and you'll miss them."

I remember dismissing that advice, because back then, an hour was an eternity and the days were measured by how quickly we could get to nap time.

But here I am, years later, planning a high school graduation party. And what do you know... the mother-in-law...she was right.

Here I am, indeed, wondering how it's possible that motherhood has come to an end so quickly– because now I have a son who will be going off to college in New York in the fall. I can't even bear to think of the day when we will be driving out east and saying goodbye in front of a dorm room. I don't even want to know what it will be like to sit down to dinner each night with an empty chair at the table. When I close my eyes, I can remember burying my nose in David's hair, drinking in the sweet scent of a newborn baby. Today, when I go to hug my teenager, my arms wrap around a body that can bench press a few hundred pounds. How is it possible that the little baby that I held in my arms just yesterday is now graduating from high school?

Just like that, eighteen years have passed by.

Yes, just like that.

(This was originally printed in the Chicago Tribune TribLocal)

Chapter 13
Looking Back

Time is a companion that goes with us on a journey. It reminds us to cherish each moment, because it will never come again. What we leave behind is not as important as how we have lived.

~ Jean Luc Picard
(yeah, we're quoting Star Trek here)

I'm nearing the end of the journey of raising my kids with my last two in high school and my oldest off to college. I've packed two decades of parenting under my belt, yet, every day continues to bring new feelings and new experiences.

In the beginning of the journey, when everything is new, sometimes it's so hard to trust your own instincts and know what to do. But throughout the whole journey, I believe there are two questions that every kid wants the answer to:

Am I loved?

Do I matter?

As parents, if we can keep the answers to those questions first and foremost in our mind as we travel on this path with our kids, those answers will guide us every step of the way.

Ten years ago, when I met Leeanne Seaver, her son Dane was several years older than David. I often turned to her for a dose of seasoned advice. Whenever I wailed to her, "What should I do?" she would gently guide me back to my instincts every time.

In one of her columns in the *Hands & Voices Communicator*, she wrote some lessons to her younger self. Lesson number one was simple:

Trust your instincts. Continue to trust your instincts. Become suspect of anyone who dismisses your concerns, or steers you away from trusting your instincts.

There were other lessons:

It's not ok to be behind—not at all ok. Don't settle.

Hold your whole family to the high standard you expect your kid to reach relative to effective communication and full access to it.

When faced with the dilemma, "should I correct his speech/language or just let this precious moment between us happen," you should always let the moment happen.

You did the best you knew how…we all do…some of where you fell short of the goal was due to circumstances beyond your control.

During a break from one of our meetings over the winter, I asked Leeanne to reflect on what she learned most from her journey of raising her son. What was the lesson which stood out on the journey?

Here's what Leeanne shared:

> "I couldn't possibly reduce the experience of raising my deaf son to a single statement expressing the most important thing I learned along the way...but as I pondered that question, it did come to me that I should just ask Dane how we did, his dad and I. He was grown and launched and well qualified to answer that question. I wondered if I even wanted to know his answer—maybe I should just wait until I was on my deathbed before asking because surely by then he wouldn't be mad about Saturday morning speech therapy any more. Or if he was, he probably wouldn't bring it up at a time like that. On the other hand, if he was still resentful about all those things that frustrated him, then I wouldn't want him to live like that his whole life. He deserved to vent, and I loved him enough to take the heat. So I asked him. Dane considered his response thoroughly before slowly answering.
>
> 'No matter what, I always knew you loved me. That was the most important thing.'
>
> Yes, I thought as I tried to swallow the lump in my throat, in the end that is the one undeniable, unchanging, non-controversial truth about this journey: love is always the most important thing."

As you progress on this journey with your child, remember Dane's words:

"You always loved me…no matter what… that was the most important thing."

Chapter 14
One Last Lesson

You didn't really think I was done, did you? I want to throw in one last lesson before you close this book. A few years back, I wrote a post for a monthly writing topic on a friend's blog. The lesson that month was: *What I Learned From Laughter.*

The lesson I'm about to share is such a profound one on the journey of raising kids—any kids! So I'm sharing it here because it is one of the most valuable life lessons I've learned.

What I Learned from Laughter

When I think about what I've learned from laughter, there's one episode in my life that stands out. When the three kids were younger, I often had days when I counted the minutes until the hubby would arrive home and provide an extra pair of eyes and hands in my quest to keep three kids in one place.

My oldest kiddo, David, was often on hurricane cycle. He would bounce from one activity to the next (like his Mom??) and leave a path of destruction in his wake. I once put the baby down for a nap and left David and Lauren parked in front of the TV so I could quickly go to the bathroom. I walked into the kitchen to find the two of them drawing wavy lines on the kitchen wall. In a matter of seconds, David had grabbed some crayons off the counter and coerced his sister into drawing artwork on the flat white builder's paint. The artwork stayed on the wall for over a year– because neither the hubby nor I could muster up enough energy to paint over the crayon.

One evening, David was a category five and my patience was long gone. I was just trying to survive long enough until the hubby arrived home so I could hand off the kid duties to him. The hubby arrived home and surveyed the toys strewn about, the lunch dishes on the table and me with the harried look on my face. He could tell it was "one of those days."

After a hurried dinner, I filled the bathtub up and went to grab towels from the other bathroom. As I walked back in, my eyes caught something floating in the bathtub.

I screamed.

It was a brand new book: ***Don't Sweat the Small Stuff*** by Richard Carlson.

I fished it out of the water, wiped as much of the wet stuff off as I could and started to cry. I sat on the toilet and the tears kept coming. Mothering three kids just two years apart had taken its toll and came crashing down on me at that moment. Just then, David came over, climbed in my lap and started hugging me.

"I love you Mommy." He hugged me again.

My eyes went back to the book and I saw the title more clearly. ***Don't Sweat the Small Stuff.***

I started to laugh.

Alternating between tears and laughter, I smiled at the irony of the whole thing.

It is now years later— the little boy has grown into a young man— but I still have the book with the warped pages stuck together. It's a reminder of that hectic time of three kids under the age of four—when I thought the day would never end and I'd never have a minute to myself. Today, the kids amuse themselves and there's a little more time for me. How quickly the time flies, how valuable that lesson of laughter is.

Don't sweat the small stuff. And remember to laugh in the process.

KAREN PUTZ GREW UP
HARD OF HEARING AND
BECAME DEAF AS A TEEN.
SHE SPENT A LOT OF TIME
WORKING WITH FAMILIES WITH
DEAF AND HARD OF HEARING
CHILDREN, PROVIDING SUPPORT
AND GUIDANCE.

WHEN HER THREE CHILDREN
BEGAN LOSING THEIR HEARING,
KAREN FIGURED SHE HAD ALL THE
ANSWERS AS A PROFESSIONAL AND
AS A DEAF PERSON.

INSTEAD, SHE DISCOVERED IT
WAS A WHOLE OTHER BALLGAME
TO NAVIGATE LIFE AS A PARENT
ON THE TWISTS AND TURNS
OF THE JOURNEY.

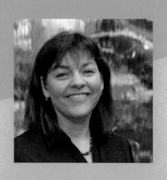

ISBN 9781479353019

90000 >

9 781479 353019